HUMANITY IN MEDICINE

THE LIFE OF PHYSICIAN DR STANLEY GOULSTON

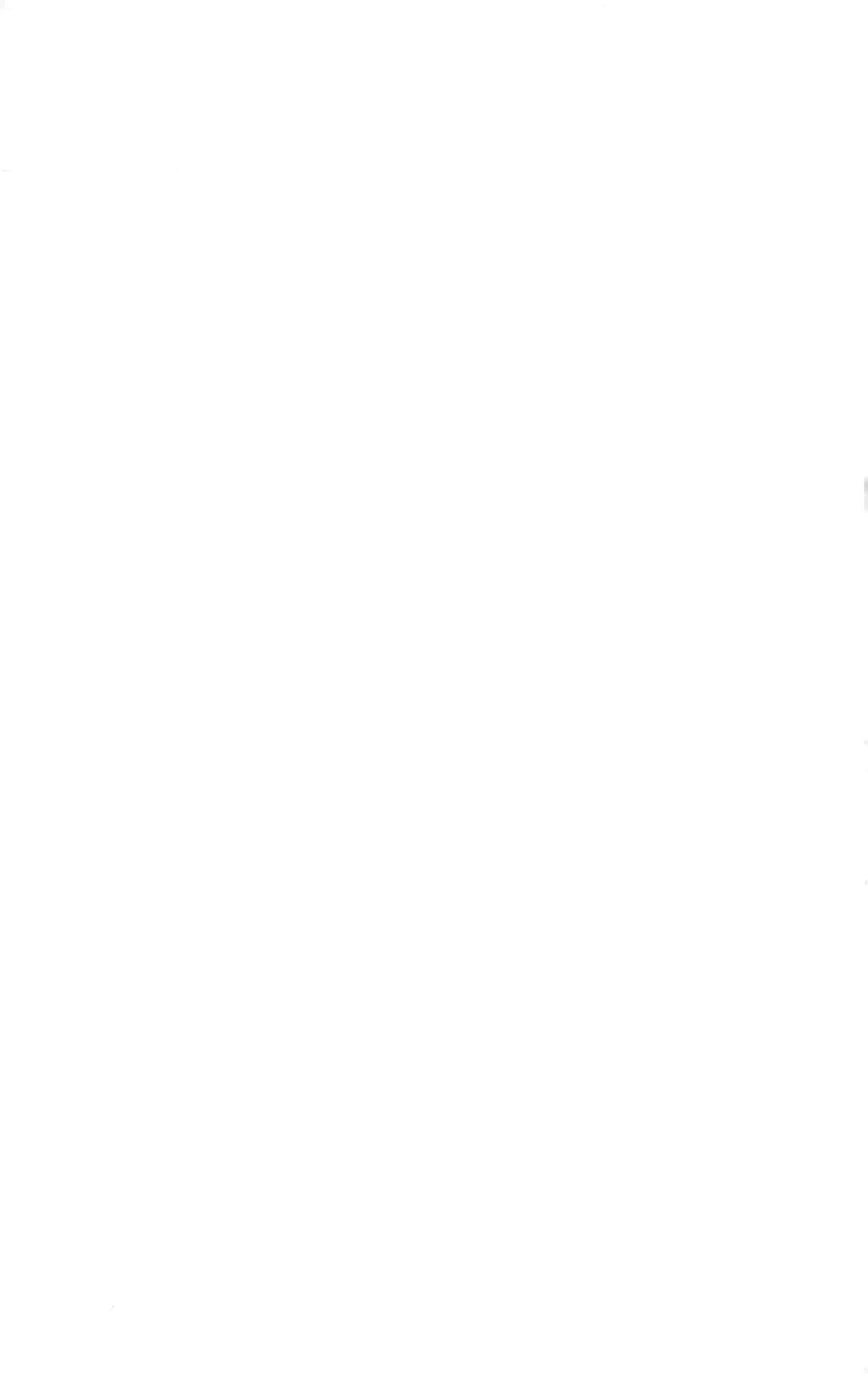

HUMANITY IN MEDICINE

THE LIFE OF PHYSICIAN DR STANLEY GOULSTON

KERRY BREEN

ARCADIA

First published 2020 by Arcadia
the general books' imprint of
Australian Scholarly Publishing Ltd
7 Lt Lothian St Nth, North Melbourne, Vic 3051
Tel: +61 3 9329 6963 / enquiry@scholarly.info / www.scholarly.info

ISBN 978-1-922454-16-4 Hardback
ISBN 978-1-922454-17-1 Paperback

Cover illustration: Portrait of Stan Goulston painted by Judy Cassab, 1976

Cover design: Wayne Saunders

Contents

Foreword

I suppose that everyone holds memories of admirable people who have become, for them, paradigms of good humanity. The Apocryphal book of Ecclesiasticus enjoins us to be grateful to physicians and to praise famous people for, among other things, 'giving counsel by their understanding' and for 'their knowledge of learning meet for the people, wise and eloquent in their instructions'. Specifically mentioned are those who 'recited verses in writing'. Of such good folk, Ecclesiasticus assures us, 'The people will tell of their wisdom, and the congregation will shew forth their praise'.

Ecclesiasticus notes that plenty of good people leave no memorial except the generations of their children and the memories of those who knew them. It is therefore very important for this biography to be written now about an extraordinary, wise, intelligent physician and teacher, a man of courage in war, of love for family and friends, of moral wisdom and broad humanity, while there are still people around whose lives were directly touched and shaped by his.

Stanley Goulston was one of the most impressive and compassionate humans I have ever met. He was reserved and self-effacing, but never remote. Shrewd in his judgement of people, he preserved a personal integrity amid the uncertainty generated by the ambitions of others, a steadiness of trust in his own values and the courage to enact them. As you read this book, you will meet someone you would most likely have wished to know. His distinguished careers as physician, researcher, teacher, professional leader, counsellor must be seen as a whole along with his heroism in war, his Judaism, his passion for the humanities (and poetry in particular), and his deep commitment to family. This was a complex man, not reducible to one label. He could deliver sound diagnosis, wise advice on matters of judgement, and light occasional verse for family celebrations and anniversaries. He fulfilled the stringent criteria that Ecclesiasticus set out to prompt the congregation to 'shew forth their praise'.

Kerry Breen's careful research brings together the multiplex strands of Stan's life. If you want to meet a human being rightly revered for the breadth of his attributes and capabilities, read on! You may come to share with us some sense of the illumination and stability that he offered to those around him and the immense affection we felt for him.

Emeritus Professor Miles Little
University of Sydney

Preface

A publisher once explained that books likely to sell well nowadays are those written by celebrities or about celebrities. If that is correct, this book will not sell well as the last claim that Sydney physician, the late Dr Stanley Goulston, would have ever made was that he was a celebrity. I suspect that if he had been approached about having his life story written, he would have rejected the idea. He may have been persuaded by the following arguments that I now use to justify this account of his life, but as he was a humble man, I cannot be sure. Fortunately his family members were persuaded and assisted me unstintingly in the writing of this account.

My arguments are general and specific. Generally, biographies are a major means by which society keeps a record of its people and its history. If thoroughly researched and well written, a biography not only portrays the life of an individual but can depict many aspects of the physical, cultural, professional and moral environment of an era. In the case of medical biographies, they can help to trace the history of medicine.

In relation to Stan Goulston, my reasons for wanting to write his story include a desire to see a modest and humble man's significant contributions to Australian medicine publicly acknowledged and recorded. He was a key player in the development of the medical specialty of gastroenterology in Australia, a role that has not yet been fully acknowledged. I make no criticism of the authors of the official history of the Gastroenterological Society of Australia, as if ever a person 'hid their light under a bushel' it was surely Goulston.

His practising life encompassed what many might say was the most remarkable fifty-year epoch in the history of medicine. His life was lived during three of the most significant dramas in Australian history: the 1919 influenza pandemic, the 1929 stock market crash leading to the Great Depression and the 1939 outbreak of World War II (with this book written – fittingly perhaps – during the fourth significant drama: the Covid-19 pandemic in 2020). His response to the outbreak of war, along with the responses of his contemporaries, should be inspirational for today's young doctors. His Army role was no more special than that of many of his contemporaries, but chance placed him at one of the most important battles of World War II and he more than played his part.

He was central to the development of specialisation in medicine at one of Australia's leading hospitals. Some might say it was 'the' leading hospital and I for one would not argue against that contention. He also led a major reform of the training of young Australian physicians and the methods by which they are assessed for fellowship of the Royal Australasian College of Physicians.

Throughout his career, he was attuned to what are now called the non-cognitive or humanistic characteristics desirable in doctors. After retiring from clinical practice, he sought to promote means of fostering these characteristics in young doctors. Of the many legacies that Stan Goulston has left for the medical profession, I hope it his wish to see more humanity in the practice of scientific medicine that receives the most consideration. His dream was to see Australian medical schools and medical educators give greater attention and adequate resources to the education of medical students and doctors in the humanities. As he once explained to a journalist, 'Science is concerned with the disease, the diagnosis, treatment and possible cure, literature with the meaning of the illness to the patient. Literature develops our sympathies and makes us feel something of what it is like to be ill or to be the relative of someone who is ill.'[1]

Acronyms

AAMC	Australian Army Medical Corps
ADEC	Australian Drug Evaluation Committee (of the Federal Department of Health)
AGH	Army General Hospital
AIF	Australian Imperial Force
CME	(career-long) continuing medical education
CMF	Citizens Military Force
CRU	Clinical Research Unit (at RPAH)
DGAMS	Director-General of Army Medical Services (UK)
FRACP	Fellowship of the Royal Australasian College of Physicians
GE Unit	Gastroenterology Unit (at RPAH)
GESA	Gastroenterological Society of Australia
GI	gastrointestinal
GPS	(Sydney) Greater Public Schools Association
JRMO	Junior Resident Medical Officer
MBBS	Bachelor of Medicine and Bachelor of Surgery
MCQs	multiple choice question examinations (of the RACP)
MRACP	Membership of the Royal Australasian College of Physicians
NCOs	non-commissioned officers

RACP	Royal Australasian College of Physicians
RACS	Royal Australasian College of Surgeons
RAP	Regimental Aid Post
RMO	Resident Medical Officer (also wartime: Regimental Medical Officer)
RPAH	Royal Prince Alfred Hospital (Sydney)
SC	Staff Corps
SGS	Sydney Grammar School
TGA	Therapeutic Goods Administration

CHAPTER 1

Family Origins and Childhood

The Goulston family has been in Australia for over 150 years. Stanley Goulston's grandfather, Hyman Goulston, came to Australia from England in 1858, aged twenty-three.[1] Hyman, son of Moses Goulston from Kabish in Poland, was born in Poland but his family migrated to London along with other Jewish refugees in the first half of the nineteenth century. Hyman was listed in the 1851 UK Census as Hyman Goldstein.

Hyman Goulston lived for a short time in Sydney, where he established a clothing and mercery store near the corner of King Street and George Street.[2] He sold that business and in 1867 moved to New Zealand, where a gold rush was creating better business opportunities. Hyman opened a clothing store in Hokitika, on the west coast of the South Island. At the height of the New Zealand gold rush, Hokitika was New Zealand's second busiest port.[3] Here Hyman became well known as 'the loser's friend' for his generous assistance to those fossickers who had failed – assistance that was noted by his children. Hyman's son and Stan's father, John Goulston, was born in Hokitika in 1869. He was the fourth child of five. John completed his schooling in New Zealand and was top of his class. He left school at the age of twelve or thirteen as he was needed to work in his father's store. With falling trade, his parents[4] decided to return to Australia in 1888.[5]

Upon return, Hyman with his four sons established clothing stores in North Sydney, Newtown and West Maitland, trading as Goulston and

Company. In 1893, Maitland was hit by a record flood of the Hunter River. Not only was that business ruined but, for two days, it was assumed that John Goulston had drowned. He had in fact been so exhausted trying to save the business that he slept for twenty-four hours. When he awoke, he found that a newspaper had announced his death.

Desperately worried for his future, John approached a local bank manager who, on a handshake, loaned the brothers and their father the money to start again. John Goulston and his descendants held accounts with that branch for the next sixty years.[6] Despite his youth, John became well known in Maitland, with help for example from the local Catholic church. He had a good tenor voice and, as well as singing in his synagogue, he sometimes sang in the Catholic church. In return, the parish priest would promote their shop at Mass with the words: 'You must go to the Goulston brothers, they are great friends of mine'.[7] It was in Maitland that John first joined the Freemasons.

In 1895, Hyman retired from business and the family partnership was dissolved.[8] The business was divided and John Goulston with his brother Solomon took over the stores in West Maitland and Newtown, while their brother Moses received the North Sydney store. With the businesses well established in Maitland and Newtown, John and Solomon expanded into Sydney, setting up another store in Brickfield Hill in central Sydney.[9] At around this time, having lived in Maitland for eight years, John moved to live in Sydney.[10] Their Brickfield Hill premises were acquired by the State Government in 1917 for the construction of Sydney's underground railway and the store was closed, leaving the brothers to focus on the Newtown business.

In 1902, John Goulston married Flora Wollff and they lived in Sydney, in Boyce Street in Glebe. Flora, born in Melbourne and into a musical family, was a talented violinist. John and Flora's first child, Olive Aroha, was born in Sydney in 1903 followed by a son, Eric Hyman, born in 1905, Edna Maud, born in 1910 and then Stanley Jack Marcus, born in Glebe in 1915. Baby Stanley was never to know or remember his mother as she died, three weeks after giving birth, of puerperal septicaemia.[11] For the next four years, John Goulston received great support from his friend, Rabbi Jacob Danglow, and the Rabbi's wife May, in caring for young Stanley and his sisters Olive and Edna and brother Eric, even though the Danglows were based in Melbourne.[12] John hired a live-in housekeeper.[13] Through these difficult years, the extended Jewish family ties helped to hold the family together. It is not known what part Olive and Edna played, if any, in caring for Stan but perhaps Eric contributed. This might help to explain the close relationship that Stan and Eric had for all their lives, despite the ten-year age difference.

Four years after the death of his first wife, John Goulston remarried. His bride was Golda Danglow,[14] the sister of his friend Jacob Danglow.[15] John was now fifty and his new wife was twenty-eight. With the marriage, the family moved from Glebe to live in Billyard Avenue, Elizabeth Bay. From this second marriage, John had two more children – a daughter, Peggy Rose, born in 1920 and a son, Roy Frank, born in 1923. As a young boy, Stan became the link between these two families, a role that was to have a considerable influence on his development and probably on his career. Stan had a good relationship with his stepmother,[16] although he never saw her as his real mother. His name for her was 'Mim' as distinct from 'Mum'. He kept in his heart a deep awareness and sense of loss of the mother he never knew. He sought older family and friends who could tell him about her, but none could satisfy his need. Every year without fail, on her yahrzeit – the date of his mother's death – he attended the synagogue to recite the Kaddish – prayers of mourning – for her.

The origin of the friendship between Rabbi Danglow and John Goulston is obscure, but it was very close and John frequently visited the Danglows in Melbourne. Jacob Danglow had been recruited from England to be the rabbi[17] at the St Kilda Synagogue in Melbourne. He was twenty-five years old and single when he arrived in 1905. A little later, his elder sister Rose followed him and for a brief time acted as his house-keeper. Jacob was a tall, athletic, handsome man who enjoyed many sports. He was academically inclined, as in addition to graduating from the London Jews' College he had studied arts at University College London and later took a Bachelor of Arts and a Master of Arts (1911) at the University of Melbourne. He spoke with a beautiful English accent and was fluent in French, German and several Arabic languages. He served his congregation for fifty-two years. He was also ecumenically inclined and played golf with Protestant and Catholic religious leaders. He served as a chaplain to the Australian Army in France in 1918 and again in World War II, now as the Senior Australian Rabbi. In 1950 he was made an Officer of the Order of the British Empire (OBE) and in 1956, a Companion of the Order of St Michael and St George (CMG). He was to become revered by the Australian Jewish community[18] and highly respected by the broader Australian society.[19]

In 1909 Jacob married May Henrietta Baruch, the daughter of Bertha Baruch (née Michaelis), a member of one of the St Kilda Synagogue's founding families. At the Danglow home, John Goulston was especially welcomed by their children – Claire, Jean and Frank. Some of the Goulston children were allowed to make the train trip to Melbourne to stay with the Danglows, with – as we shall see – one significant long-term consequence.

John Goulston proved to be a successful businessman, so much so that he retired young, relying on his knowledge of investing. To have money available to invest, he rented a home instead of buying one. However, when the Great Depression arrived in 1929, he was ruined and had to go back to work. In his second career, he served on the Board of Greater Union Theatres from 1934 to 1961 and became vice-chairman. His involvement began as an activist shareholder who regularly attended the annual general meetings and this led to his being elected as a director. He had never been interested in movies but now went to the State Theatre every Saturday night with his wife, no matter what film was being shown.[20] He also served as President of the Retail Traders Association[21] and as a board member for a number of companies.

With the onset of the Great Depression, John Goulston was under financial pressure and at one point suffered a nervous breakdown.[22] His eldest son Eric, now a young doctor, was deeply concerned for his father's well-being and phoned the Danglows for advice. On hearing this news,

May Danglow insisted that John come to Melbourne to stay with them and be cared for. Within a few months, he was back in Sydney restored to good health.[23]

John Goulston rose to a prominent and respected place in Sydney's commercial world and among the Sydney Jewish community. He served on the Board of the Great Synagogue[24] for many years and was its President from 1932 to 1936 and again from 1944 to 1945. He loved the synagogue's choir and each year would host a dinner for them at his own expense. He was elected a life member of the synagogue in 1939. He was active in many Jewish organisations in Sydney, including the Jewish Welfare Society, the Australian Jewish Historical Society and the Jewish Education Board. He was the foundation Secretary of the Jewish War Memorial. He played a major role in the establishment of the New South Wales Jewish Advisory Board, which was later to become the Board of Deputies.[25] He was a strong supporter of Jewish youth and donated a prize to be awarded to the best one-act play mounted by young people at the Annual Drama Festival. In a history of the Great Synagogue written in 2008, it was noted that 'his whole family has always been prominent in the Great Synagogue'.[26]

That John Goulston took his family to the Great Synagogue regularly is attested to by his son Stan's contribution to the 2008 history. Stan wrote for the book a long contribution entitled 'Precious and Vivid Memories'.[27] He recalled the beauty of the building during Friday night services and the unbearable heat in summer. He also recalled Rabbi Francis Cohen as being rather severe and not allowing children on the bimah – the raised area of the synagogue with seating and standing-room for participants and with a reading desk for prayers and for Torah (Old Testament) and Haftorah (The Prophets) readings – with the result that at their Bar Mitzvah, the children regarded this 'with awe and fear'. He noted that in those days, there were no Jewish day schools so religious classes were held in the synagogue after the Sabbath service and that the Hebrew classes held on Sunday mornings were unpopular.[28]

John and his second wife raised their children in the Anglo-Orthodox tradition of Judaism. The Great Synagogue rabbis were recruited from

England where Jewish religious practices were more relaxed, in line with Ashkenazi custom. One of his granddaughters stated that, as a result, 'we grew up in the Ashkenazi tradition with a bit of Sephardic thrown in'.[29] John's second wife, Golda, ran a kosher household but was flexible when away from home.[30] Golda was described by Stan as a passive woman, 'which suited his father but they got on well'.[31]

John Goulston was also an active Freemason and was Grand Master of the Grand Lodge of New South Wales for several years. He later insisted that his sons join the lodge. This they did but they were never active members. From the reminiscences of his granddaughters, John Goulston was perceived as a formal man and an authoritarian father who expected his children to do exactly as he told them to do.[32] Despite his formal side, he was comfortable mixing in any circle. He was faithful to his religion and dutiful in attending the synagogue.[33] John was rigid in some of his attitudes, as was possibly shown when he refused to give his second daughter, Edna, permission to marry a non-Jew.[34] He successfully instilled a sense of public duty in his six children, as was seen when World War II broke out. In 1943, four of his six offspring and his son-in-law were in the military; his daughter Edna was a Second Officer with the Women's Royal Australian Naval Service (WRANS) and three of the men were Majors.[35]

In July 1939, John Goulston was selected to represent the Grand Lodge of New South Wales and its Grand Master, Lord Gowrie, at the installation of the Duke of Kent as Grand Master of the Grand Lodge of English Freemasons. The ceremony was performed by King George V, a Past Grand Master of the Grand Lodge, in the presence of fourteen thousand Freemasons. For John Goulston, this involved a round-the-world trip, first to the UK and then to the USA – a trip that was reported in a Sydney Jewish newspaper.[36] His journey to the UK was by flying-boat, an onerous trip that began from Rose Bay and involved twenty-three stops.

In London, after the installation ceremony, he was presented to the King, was a guest of the House of Commons and attended a banquet given by the Lord Mayor of London. While in London, he met many Jewish 'leaders of commercial and social life'.[37] He had also been asked by the

Great Synagogue to choose a new rabbi and he selected Rabbi Porush, who had been recommended to him by the Jews' College.[38]

John Goulston then sailed on the *Queen Mary* to New York and there, and in San Francisco, he met with leaders of the Jewish communities. He returned safely to Sydney by ship, arriving in early October 1939 – a voyage made potentially hazardous by the declaration of war at the beginning of September.

Although much of his community service was to his Jewish community, he was also active in many other spheres. As mentioned, he served as President of the Retail Traders Association. He chaired a group that settled a major New South Wales railway dispute in 1917,[39] chaired a Greek Relief Fund, and he was a governor of the Royal Prince Alfred Hospital and the Balmain Hospital. A ward in the Balmain Hospital was named in his honour for his generosity.[40] He played a leading role in the formation of the Kolling Research Institute at Royal North Shore Hospital, through his trusted association with the Kolling family. He was also a member of the Sydney Cricket Club for fifty years.

He was honoured in a number of ways. His Freemason's Lodge commissioned his portrait in 1948. The portrait, by artist Joseph Wolinski,[41] was hung in the Masonic Temple in Castlereagh Street. Wolinski painted a second portrait of Goulston, in informal attire, and Wolinski entered this in the 1948 Archibald Prize and was a finalist that year.[42] John Goulston was made a Member of the Order of the British Empire (MBE) in 1958 for services to the community. On his ninetieth birthday, he received a telegram of congratulations from Prime Minister Menzies.[43]

John Goulston was determined that where possible his children would get a tertiary education – something he had missed out on, although he had long harboured a desire to become a doctor.[44] He succeeded, as five of his six children received a tertiary education: three medical practitioners, a pharmacist and a scientist.[45] He also impressed on his children the importance of having a good name, developed through honesty, hard work and thinking of others.[46]

As might be imagined, John's second marriage and his wide outside interests had a significant impact on Stan's childhood. However, it was basically a happy childhood, one lived in a secure environment. Being the youngest of John's children with Flora, Stan even as a boy appreciated that he was the 'bridge' between the children of the two marriages. He was well aware that his elder sisters made life difficult for his stepmother. He developed great respect[47] for her and, as he grew older, he sought to support her as much as he could.[48] He developed a special bond with his elder brother Eric and related well to his younger siblings, Peggy and Roy. He saw little of his busy father but his stepmother, who was always at home, was an ever-present part of his life. Her only outings were to the movies with her husband every Saturday evening and her attendance at synagogue. She was a good cook and on Sundays, when her cook had the day off,[49] made pancakes as a treat for her children.

While the family always had a maid and a cook, John Goulston never became a wealthy man, perhaps because he was so involved in community activities. Many middle-class families employed home help in Australia before World War II and this was not an indicator of great wealth. Few married women sought outside employment and a clear separation of the role of the wife at home versus the husband at work was the norm. John Goulston rented for most of his married life and only once owned a home. He happily used public transport[50] and did not buy a motor-car until late in life.

Although Stan's father had four siblings, these uncles and an aunt were not a large part of Stan's upbringing. The family connections were much stronger with his stepmother's Melbourne family.

Stan recalled that as a child he felt intimidated by his authoritarian father. For example, at one point he badly needed new shoes but was afraid to tell his father. He was aware that younger brother Roy was treated differently and described him as confident and 'thoroughly spoilt, completely indulged'. He was heedful that his father expected all his children to study hard. His father did not participate in family holidays.[51] It was only when Stan himself became a father and John Goulston had retired that a closer understanding between them grew. The roles then were reversed, as it was his father who was warning him that he was working too hard.[52] In old age, Stan reflected that 'parts of my life when I was a child were not good' and added 'I think that it was partly my fault'.[53]

Early in his childhood, Stan took an interest in gardening; he grew pansies to give to his teacher. The family home in Elizabeth Bay had sufficient space and soil in the front yard and here he grew vegetables. At times he was a solitary child and played games that he invented, often with marbles; because he played against himself, he always won. The house had a large brick wall where he could practise tennis on his own. In 1930 when he was thirteen, he won a red certificate for a letter published in the junior section of the Sydney *Sun* that described a new game he had invented, called 'breaking the stick'.[54] At the age of fourteen, he was submitting poems to the same newspaper.

As well as at times being a solitary child, Stan was also sensitive, alert to the interchanges between the people around him and what they might be feeling, especially the possibility that somebody might be hurt. Late in life he was to reflect that perhaps this 'was not good for me ... I was much too sensitive'.[55] He deemed himself also to have been a very serious child, stating 'nothing was light for me'.[56]

While secure, Stan's childhood was not without its dramas. His earliest memories were of people in the street near his Glebe home wearing masks in the 1919 influenza pandemic. He later learned that at about the time he was born and his mother died, his brother Eric and sister Olive had become ill with typhoid fever and scarlet fever. He was also told that, at that point, he was being wet-nursed and the woman engaged for the task was not a success; Stan's father apparently was critical that the wet-nurse fed her own baby first.[57] These were stressful times for his father. Other childhood memories included the views from their Elizabeth Bay home across Sydney Harbour and hearing lions roaring at night at the Sydney Zoo on the north side of the harbour.

As Flora Goulston was involved in music and played the violin well, her children were encouraged to learn a musical instrument.[58] This continued after her death and Stan was allocated the violin, in honour of his late mother. At the age of six he began classes with some local nuns and these continued for five years or so. However, he never enjoyed this and preferred to 'muck up' with his younger brother or to listen to the gramophone instead of practising. He at times skipped lessons without telling his family and, as a result, 'got into a great deal of trouble' with his father.[59] Finally he was rescued from this unhappy situation by Aunt Martha Wollff, his birth mother's sister, also a talented violinist. As a ten-year-old on his first visit to Melbourne, Stan was asked by Aunt Martha to bring his violin with him. Soon after his arrival, Aunt Martha insisted that they play together. She must have quickly decided that Stan did not have much talent, as she commented that 'Kreisler has no need to be worried'.[60] Luckily Stan's dislike of playing the violin did not prevent him from developing a love of music.

He enjoyed his visits to Melbourne, staying with the Danglow family two or three times when he was fifteen and sixteen. He was a natural and interested observer of family dynamics, in his own family and at the Danglows. He spent time with his Uncle Jacob in his study on many evenings and observed that his Uncle 'would never decide on anything without asking Aunty May's advice'.[61]

Tooth decay was common in Australia then and little dental care was available. Stan was no exception. At the age of fourteen, he needed major work done on his teeth. His elder brother Eric had recently graduated as a doctor and was working in a general practice at Crows Nest, where he and his young wife lived above the surgery. It was arranged that a dentist would come to the surgery and that Eric would give the required anaesthetic. Stan stayed with his brother and sister-in-law for a few days to recover.

An unhappier encounter with medical care as a young boy was also recalled. His father arranged for a well-known surgeon to remove Stan's tonsils. Stan found the experience 'terrifying' but the aspect that still angered him seventy years later was that the surgeon never spoke a word to him, before or after the operation.

Stan's father, John Goulston, died in Sydney in 1961 at the age of ninety-two. Stan's stepmother, Golda, had died in 1952 at the age of sixty-one.

John Goulston was honoured by a state funeral held at the Great Synagogue attended by a thousand mourners. Rabbi Porush delivered the eulogy and drew attention to Goulston's role as a leader of the Jewish community, his championing of Australian Jewish people and his broader service to the general community. In a tribute to him published in November 1961, it was said: 'The name of John Goulston will … in the future be cherished with respect, and his memory will be upheld in a spirit of admiration and honour for a man who has deserved well of all the branches of our community'.[62]

CHAPTER 2

Youthful Years

Young Stanley Goulston's formal education began when he was enrolled in a nearby private primary school known as Edgecliff Preparatory School, which was then an informal feeder for Sydney Grammar School.[1] His elder brother and his two elder sisters had attended the State School system for their primary education.[2] Stan enjoyed the Edgecliff School and won prizes for his efforts. Although in a small minority as a Jewish boy, he never sensed any maltreatment or discrimination at school.[3] His enjoyment of sport began here and grew further when, at thirteen, he moved up to secondary school.

That was also the year of his Bar Mitzvah, a very important event in his life[4] and one that he recalled clearly. He was nervous but proud to be a Cohen, a group ('Cohanim' in Hebrew) regarded in modern orthodox Jewish tradition as the descendants of Old Testament Jewish priests. As a member of this group, which continues to have religious status and ceremonial responsibility, Stan was to be called up to read the last part of the Torah (Old Testament) in Hebrew. His part, of ten minutes or so duration, included a point where he had to sing some key words and then the choir joined in – a choir[5] that included his elder sister Olive, which would have increased his feelings of pride. Later he recognised that the event 'helped a great deal in one's development'. Nowadays, a Bar Mitzvah is usually followed by a party but in 1928 an 'at home' was held at John and Golda's residence on the weekend, and family and friends dropped in to pay their respects.[6] As an additional reward, Stan, along with four of his friends, was taken by elder brother Eric to see a musical comedy.

His father expected Stan to attend class at the synagogue on Sundays and he attended regularly for a number of years. Here he was taught Jewish history and was supposed to learn Hebrew. He resented the class, primarily because it meant that his whole weekend was taken up with religious duties. He did, however, enjoy the teaching of a Russian man who related stories of interest from Europe. As part of his religious duties, Stan recalled that as a boy on Yom Kippur (the Day of Atonement) he and his family would have a meal at 5 p.m. in preparation for fasting that lasted twenty-four hours. After the meal, they would walk together the long distance from Elizabeth Bay to the Great Synagogue in the city.

During his school years, Stan was very close to elder brother Eric – a bond that lasted a lifetime. Eric was now studying medicine at the University of Sydney. As one small example of this bond, each evening before he went to bed, Stan would take a cup of cocoa to Eric where he was studying in his room. Eric would drop what he was doing and chat with his little brother for ten minutes while they both drank their cocoas. Given the ten-year age difference between Stan and Eric and the remoteness of their father, perhaps Eric then was also a father figure for this sensitive young boy.

In 1929, Stan moved from Edgecliff School to enter Sydney Grammar School (SGS) in Form II – Year Eight in modern parlance. This school, established in 1857, is a private non-sectarian institution which has never had a religious basis. The school is a member of the prestigious Sydney Greater Public Schools Association (GPS).[7] Although Stan's father left school at a young age, he was determined that his children would have a good education and, if possible, attend university; in this aim, he was successful.[8] In that era, there were no Jewish private schools so a non-sectarian prestigious and accessible private school was an obvious choice. For young Stan, it was always likely to happen as his brother Eric had attended SGS ten years earlier. It is a boys-only school and in the year that Stan first attended the total enrolment was around 600 students. Of these, 180 were 'new boys', although some of those joined the school in higher forms.

That year, the new boys were told by the headmaster: '[Y]ou belong to a great institution, one that has won for itself in past years praise and respect from every quarter … from now on Grammar will be judged, for good or bad, according to your appearance and general conduct whenever you are wearing the school uniform'.[9] One small piece of evidence about the attitudes that the school inculcated into its students was the impressive number of Old Collegians who later enlisted to serve the nation in World War II.[10]

The school leaders during Goulston's five years at SGS were alert to the social upheavals beyond Australia's shores, especially the rise of fascism, and the boys were not sheltered from these developments. At the school assembly and prize-giving in late 1929, the boys were addressed by the New South Wales Governor, Sir Dudley de Chair, and his speech was reported in the *Sydney Morning Herald* on 14 December[11] of that year. He was reported as saying:

> One of the chief dangers of democracy was the tendency to level men down to a standard of mediocrity – to adapt the chain to its weakest link. Unless this tendency was actively combated, there was always a fear that when a crisis had to be faced, there would be no man to deal with it.

Being a formal occasion, the headmaster, Mr Dettman, was in no position to debate this point of view, with its fascist tones. It is noteworthy therefore that at the same event a year later (in front of the new State Governor, Sir Philip Game), the headmaster appeared to respond to the previous Governor's remarks of the year before. Now the same newspaper quoted Dettman[12] as saying:

> Amusing and unanswerable attacks upon democracy are as old as the poet Aristophanes, but the unalienable and blessed

> fact remains that a system of democratic government does leave the mass of the people under the distinct impression that they really govern themselves – surely an enormous gain and a great contribution to happiness and contentment.

He went on to explain his school's philosophy in education and sport. It seems clear from this quality of leadership that Stanley Goulston's education was in good hands.

During Stan's time at SGS, Australia was affected by the Great Depression. The school experienced a drop in enrolments and a consequent negative impact on its budget. However, for the boys who stayed on, school life was little changed. That was not the case at home for the Goulstons, as Stan's father was badly affected by the Depression.

Stan greatly enjoyed his years at SGS and retained a warm feeling for the school throughout his life.[13] The record of his involvement in school activities shows that he wholeheartedly embraced the wide range of sporting and other activities on offer – including football, cricket, tennis, boxing, rifle shooting, a debating club and a camera club.[14] The school also had a cadet corps but the corps was struggling for numbers. In his first year, Stan entered the boxing tournament but lost his first round bout. He played in football (rugby union), cricket and tennis teams but without great distinction. In 1931 he was a member of the 7th SGS Football Team, of which 'Bassar, Davis, Heighway, Goulston and Wood were the shock troops'. In the same year, he was a member of the 4th Cricket Team and top-scored with 30 runs in a losing side against The Kings School. That year he also represented the 'School' (i.e., the day students) in the annual tennis match against the 'House' (i.e., the boarders); he lost his singles match 5–7 in a close-fought encounter. Later, as a university student, he was to find his *métier* in field hockey.

It was fortunate that Stan enjoyed sport, as it had a big place at the school. Participation was assured by placing virtually every boy in a team.[15] The headmaster in his annual address to students and parents never failed to mention success in sport. The SGS magazine, *The Sydneian*, issued three times per year, also placed a great emphasis on sporting achievements. In Stan's first year at the school, there was great rejoicing as SGS won both the GPS Football Premiership and the GPS Athletics Carnival. In that year, he may have joined his classmates to watch the First Eleven Cricket Team, hoping to see performances as remarkable as those reported for 1928 when the team's vice-captain and star batsman was Alan McGilvray, who went on to become one of Australia's most respected cricket broadcasters.[16]

Later in life, Goulston recalled his terrible conflict of conscience when trying to choose between his commitment to attend the Great Synagogue with his father on a Saturday morning or joining his school mates in sporting teams.[17] In his first year, when he was preparing for his Bar Mitzvah, most of the matches were in the morning. He recognised that he may have been embarrassing his father at the synagogue but still resorted to subterfuge by only announcing a sporting commitment at the last minute, leaving the dilemma with his father. Most often, his father would send him off to sport, saying that if you have been selected, you must not let the school down.

Stan equally applied himself to his school work. In his first year at the school, he won the Herbert Webb Memorial Prize, awarded for the student who has shown the greatest improvement during the year but has missed out on other prizes.[18] His prize was presumably a book, for in the same issue of the school magazine that listed all the prize-winners that year, a student had a letter published bemoaning the books that were given for prizes and arguing for the boys to have a say in what titles were chosen!

In 1930 Stan passed his Intermediate Certificate[19] examinations, receiving an A in English and in History and a B in Mathematics I, Latin and Chemistry. He later recalled that across New South Wales, the overall results of the Intermediate Certificate examinations that year were deemed to be poor. Letters appeared in the Sydney newspapers attributing this to the fact that the cohort were 'war babies' born around the time of Gallipoli and that their mothers had been affected by this. Yet as he pointed out, this theory seemed to be disproved when the cohort's efforts in the Leaving Certificate were back where they should be.[20]

In 1931, he earned credits in science and history. In 1932, his Leaving

Certificate results were excellent, with first-class honours in English, an A in Ancient History and Bs in Latin, French, Mathematics I, Mathematics II and Chemistry. He shared the Freeman Meeks Memorial Prize in English with E.L. Davis. We have no way of knowing what would be equivalent results today, but out of sixty-one boys from SGS who sat for the Leaving Certificate, only four others received first-class honours in any subject and Stan was the only student out of seventeen who got an A for Ancient History. The majority of boys took four or five subjects in Leaving, while Stan took eight standard and two honours subjects. He was one of eight boys from the school who gained exhibitions, enabling free entry to Sydney University. When the state-wide Order of Merit was announced a few weeks later, he was surprised to find himself very close to the top of 30,000 students.[21] The school had a policy of encouraging all students to do a second year of the Leaving class but Stan opted to take up his university place immediately.

Late in his last year at the school, Stan had his first poem published in *The Sydneian*. He titled it 'At Watson's Bay'.[22] The poem read:

> O beacon! O dazzling brightness!
> O fading light!
> Flooding the waters, retreating
> Like a falling star,
> Swift and glittering.
> O star! O brilliance!
>
> Shall it be so with me?
> Does my future gleam forth in sparkling youth?
> But – for how long?
> Must I also dim and pass into night?

At the end of the 1932–33 Sydney summer, Stan Goulston commenced his studies at the University of Sydney to become a doctor. This was then a six-year course. His elder brother had already graduated as a doctor[23] and now was in general practice at Crows Nest. Late in his life, Stan acknowledged that he chose to study medicine primarily because of Eric's influence and the admiration he held for his brother.[24] His brother was to remain his closest friend and was a mentor and role model.

As a new medical graduate, brother Eric did not lack self-confidence. Stan recalled that Eric removed the tonsils of his younger brother, Roy, when Roy was around seven or eight years old. The surgery took place on the kitchen table while Stan took Roy's mother for a walk in a local park. Dr Eric Goulston became a pioneering paediatric surgeon at the Royal Alexandra Hospital for Children and was also a general surgeon for adult patients at Royal North Shore Hospital. He was on the staff of both hospitals for thirty years. He served as a medical officer in the Army during World War II, with duties in North Africa, Greece, the Pacific theatre and on a hospital ship. When retirement from the Royal Alexandra Hospital for Children and the Royal North Shore Hospital had to be taken at the age of sixty, he took on the task of Foundation Professor of Surgery at the Medical School of Haile Selassie University at Addis Ababa in Ethiopia. Eric's interesting life deserves its own biography. A published summary is given as an appendix to this book.[25]

Whether there were other factors, conscious or subconscious, in Stan's choice of career we cannot know but perhaps the sad death of his mother soon after giving birth to him may have been an influence. He was also aware of family expectations, as there were several doctors in his extended family.[26] He was initially torn between studying literature and studying medicine. That this was a difficult decision for him was evidenced years later by what he chose to do after retiring from medical practice.

During the medical course, he lived at home with his father and stepmother at Elizabeth Bay. He was well aware that without the exhibition that he had won, he would have been unable to go to university. He was also aware of his father's expectation of hard work as a student and he did not disappoint him. To support himself to a certain extent, he took on various jobs during the long summer vacations. The Elizabeth Bay house was not large and Goulston occupied a small dark room to the rear of the house, which had a window that looked out at the brick wall of the house next door. Here for six years he spent many long hours of study.

In the first year of his Bachelor of Medicine and Bachelor of Surgery (MBBS) course, the subjects studied included chemistry, physics, biology and zoology. Goulston did well, passing with a Credit while his contemporaries from SGS, Davis and Dakin, were awarded Distinctions. In his second year, Goulston and Dakin were noted to have passed while Davis got a Credit. The correspondent for *The Sydneian* had no information about Goulston's performance in the third year of the course but reported that in fourth year, Goulston and Davis got 'good passes'.

In his first three years, Goulston played no sport at university but in fourth year, he found time for this. Although he had played cricket and football at school, at university his chosen sport was hockey. He had never played it before but found it an ideal sport for him. He compared its strategy and field positions to soccer but noted that it could be a dangerous game. This was especially so in the lower grades where skills in using a hockey stick and keeping the ball low were less well developed. Fortunately he was talented and soon was playing left wing in Sydney University's senior team. He chose this playing spot 'cannily' as he knew that he was fast over a short distance and that it was not a popular spot because one had to learn to hit backwards.[27] In 1936, as a fourth-year medical student, he was selected in the University Hockey Team and competed in the Intervarsity Carnival, that year hosted by the University of Melbourne. He was once selected in the New South Wales state team but for reasons unknown, the team did not play a game. In his fifth year of the course, he was elected secretary of the University Hockey Club. He was acknowledged for his canny choice of position and for his ability, as in 1937 he was awarded a blue for hockey by the University. This award came with a special blazer which he treasured, but it was stolen when he left clothes on Manly Beach one day.

The study pressure of the medical course left little time for cultural activities despite his declared interest in music and literature, but he was writing poetry during those years.

What was happening socially for young Stan Goulston? In his last years at school, he was spending holiday time in Melbourne with his Uncle Jacob Danglow (the brother of his stepmother) and Jacob's wife, Aunty May. He was fond of them both, but especially of Aunty May.[28] He loved to sit in his uncle's study and observe him in his reading. The Danglows had three children – Claire, Jean and Frank. Jean was Stan's age. They were for a time just 'cousins'[29] with whom to play but, at the age of seventeen, a romance blossomed between Jean and Stan. This was to be a long-distance romance – one maintained over the next seven years by letters, phone calls and occasional interstate visits by train. The depth of Stan's feeling is seen in this poem that he wrote as a third-year medical student in 1935, titled 'Jean, Aged Seventeen':

A foreign urge to achieve
Looking with wondrous eyes
Into unknown beauty,
A sense of deep comfort
A longing when she is away
Deeper than understanding

A sudden catch at seeing her unexpected
Joy when her eyes smile, a sense
Of completeness in her presence.

Laugh at the world, its fakes and fallacies
Its insincerity, cruelty, hatred,
Drink in the blue of the sea and the sky
The cry of the cricket, the swoop of the gull,

All beauty and fineness are yours
With the love of a friend.

Their romance was to last over seventy years, broken only by Jean's death.

For the clinical years of the medical course, Stan was based at the

Royal Prince Alfred Hospital (RPAH) in Camperdown, adjacent to the campus of the University of Sydney. His commitment to hockey did not interfere with his studies: his fifth-year results in 1937 were very good as he was awarded a Distinction. His final year, 1938, passed quickly and his examination results were excellent. He was awarded a Credit for his final-year examinations and was ranked fourth in the class for that year. Overall for the medical course he was awarded second-class honours, graduated in eighteenth place[30] and easily won a prized residency post at the RPAH.

At graduation, he wrote a prayer for himself that is remarkable for the maturity and thoughtfulness it demonstrates. It reads as follows:

> I pray for knowledge, for an intellect far greater than its present value, for insight to discriminate, for judgement and a balanced mind. I pray for knowledge in all culture but particularly the culture of healing. I pray for a sixth sense & personal confidence. I pray for an appreciation of all things fine and beautiful – art & literature, trees & flowers, grace & rhythm, poetry & particularly, music.
>
> If the knowledge I pray for is above my present ability I pray for energy & willpower to eventually reach a state when such knowledge may be attained, for faith in myself & pledge myself, if ever acquired, to use such art wholly for the lessening of human suffering.
>
> I pray for full friendship, to give & receive absolute trust.
>
> If ever gained I was to lose these things then might I lose appreciation of poetry & literature first, then understanding of grace & rhythm, then colour & beauty, if you will, all knowledge of Medicine, but not friendship, for without it nothing can be accomplished & without it I am useless on this earth.

On 3 January 1939, at the age of twenty-three, he commenced his appointment as Junior Resident Medical Officer (JRMO) and lived full-time at the hospital for the next fifteen months. He quickly settled into the hospital routine. He and the other twenty-one junior residents were poorly paid[31] but were provided with free accommodation, meals and laundry. Stan was not concerned about his income, as he believed that he was 'getting the best medical education you could get'. He felt that as young doctors they were valued and respected, noting that the Medical Superintendent, Dr Herbert Schlink, knew the name of every one of them. Each night at midnight, resident doctors were expected to do a brief ward round to check on the patients under their care. In his JRMO year, he spent four months in a medical rotation in the general medical unit run by Dr John Halliday, four months in a surgical unit rotation and four months of other duties, including staffing the Casualty Department. There were no external rotations to other hospitals, urban or rural.

His early experience of hospital medicine was about to be interrupted by a major event: the outbreak of World War II.

CHAPTER 3

Joining the Army

During Goulston's last years at school and during his six years as a medical student, Australia had experienced the Great Depression and had seen the evolution of fascism in Europe. In Australia, unemployment peaked at around 30 per cent in the early 1930s and the economy had not fully recovered when Goulston finished his medical course in November 1938. As a Jew, he would have been aware of the manner in which Jewish people in Germany and Austria were being treated by Hitler and he would have noted the Jewish refugees already arriving in Sydney.

In 1938, Australia was very different to the Australia of 2020. The population was only seven million people. Australians were strongly attached to the British Empire. Their passports were British. They celebrated Empire Day every 24 May with bonfires and fireworks.[1] After the Armistice of World War I, the government had greatly reduced the size of the Armed Forces.[2] Psychologically and in practice, Australians believed that the presence of the British and the Royal Navy at Singapore provided all the protection needed.

As they were part of the British Empire, Australians were unsurprised when, just hours after Britain had declared war with Germany, Australia's Prime Minister, Robert Menzies, announced on national radio on Sunday evening, Father's Day, 3 September 1939, 'It is my melancholy duty to inform you officially ... that Australia is also at war'. Historians tell us that the announcement of Menzies did not have an immediate impact in Australia. The loss of the lives of 60,000 Australian men in World War I was fresh in the minds of most citizens. There was no initial rush to enlist in the Forces. This changed when news arrived that Paris had been occupied in June 1940. Menzies' news did have an impact on the junior doctors working at Royal Prince Alfred Hospital (RPAH) and in other hospitals in Sydney. Goulston was one who sought to enlist early. Eventually, all 140 of his fellow University of Sydney medical graduates would enlist.[3] By the war's end, over one million men and women of Australia had served in the Armed Forces.

Goulston first tried to enlist in the Australian Navy but was told that he was not needed. At the end of his 1939 resident year, he successfully enlisted[4] in the Australian Army but was informed that he would not be called up until required. Accordingly, he began work again at RPAH as a second-year Resident Medical Officer. His call-up came in April 1940. He imagined that he would probably be asked to serve in an Army hospital under supervision and would, in effect, be continuing his training as a junior doctor. This was not to be.[5]

Prior to the declaration of war, Australia had only a small regular army backed up by a part-time militia or Citizens Military Force (CMF) – the equivalent today of the Army Reserve – of 37,000 men. It was a militia that was poorly equipped and not battle-ready.[6] A new force, to be named the 2nd Australian Imperial Force (2nd AIF) – the 1st AIF having been the army that went to Gallipoli and France in World War I – was hastily assembled and partly trained in Australia. The first members of this new force, the 6th Division, left Sydney by ship on 10 January 1940, bound for Palestine where their training continued and the men were exposed to even tougher training for desert warfare. On 5 May 1940, two more battalions left Australia, headed for Britain.

The occupation of Paris triggered an additional flood of volunteers in Australia so that by the end of July, 82,000 new recruits had enlisted.[7] There was no lack of volunteers and conscription was never an issue.[8] While no soldiers were conscripted into the Australian Army for overseas service,[9] legislation (the *National Security Act*) was passed in 1939 to enable the conscription of men to the CMF for home defence and the conscription of doctors. However, only volunteer doctors could be sent overseas.[10] In addition, in Britain and in Australia, the services of the ships and the crews of the merchant navy could be commandeered by the Armed Forces.[11] For the young men who enlisted, the motives varied but included a desire to see if they could match the feats of their fathers at Gallipoli and in France in 1914–1918, as well as the reality of better pay and job security. The Great Depression had severely affected Australia between 1929 and 1933. Even by the time that war broke out, the Australian economy had not fully recovered. Thus employment in the Armed Forces was attractive to many who were struggling to find satisfactory work.

When called up in April 1940, Goulston was immediately appointed a Captain attached to the Australian Army Medical Corps and undertook brief Medical Corps training. The content of this training can be surmised from a 1943 description of the role of the Regimental Medical Officer[12] where the emphasis was on the assessment of fitness for duty of the soldiers, and not on their care when ill or seriously injured. Also emphasised were the need for good relationships with other officers and the important role to be played in the maintenance of sanitation and hygiene.

When that introductory training was completed, Goulston was surprised to find himself allocated to the AIF 2nd/1st Pioneer Battalion,[13] which had been established on paper on 1 May 1940, with Lieutenant Colonel P.E. Macgillicuddy as its commanding officer. The name 'Pioneer Battalion' was inherited from the First World War, although its origin is unclear. Regardless it was an unusual battalion in that its troops needed to be trained and equipped to act as infantry (i.e., to fight) when required but also to have the knowledge and skills to undertake engineering tasks. These tasks included building and camouflaging obstacles and defence posts, repairing roads and bridges, restoring communication lines, and planning and building defences against bombardment. Some of the battalion staff were also trained in defusing bombs. Eventually four Pioneer Battalions were formed but Goulston's was the first.

On account of the need for skills and life experience that would allow this specialised battalion to be prepared for war quickly, the average age of the men allocated to the Pioneers was nearer to forty than thirty[14] – a factor that may have altered the medical work ahead for Goulston. Through its possession of these additional skills, the battalion was never fixed to one division of the Army and, over time, found itself attached to the 6th, 7th and 9th Divisions.

Towards the end of Goulston's introductory training, a rumour circulated among the men that it was likely they would be sent overseas shortly after their training was completed. Goulston was by now engaged to his childhood sweetheart, Jean Danglow.[15] On hearing this rumour, he approached his commanding officer and asked if the rumour was true. On being told that it was, he immediately asked if he could get special leave to get married.[16] The officer replied, 'You can have a week off from today'.

That same day, a Wednesday, Goulston telephoned his future mother-in-law, May Danglow, to tell her of their plans. May did not hesitate to agree to make all the necessary arrangements.[17] She moved with great haste and even managed to have an announcement of the marriage appear in two major Melbourne newspapers[18] on the day of the wedding, as well as attending to many other details. Stan, his parents and other family members, as well as fiancée Jean who was in Sydney at that time, travelled to Melbourne on Friday by the night train. Not long after their arrival, the Goulstons joined the Danglow family as guests for lunch at the home of close friends, Lucie and Reuben Hallenstein. At the lunch, when a guest suggested that it was bad luck for the bride to see the groom ahead of the wedding that evening, Lucie Hallenstein snorted 'stuff and nonsense'.[19]

Jean and Stan were married at 8 p.m. on Saturday 25 May 1940 at the St Kilda Synagogue, with Rabbi Danglow presiding. It rained during the afternoon but not for the wedding. A teenage family friend[20] who came to the synagogue to see her first wedding was able, in 2020, to describe the beautiful bride as 'floating down the aisle' where the groom was waiting looking resplendent in his Army uniform. A small reception of around twenty-five guests followed at the Danglow home. After one night at

Menzies Hotel, the newlyweds set off on a brief honeymoon. They had been loaned a small Vauxhall car and used the remaining few days to motor back to Sydney. They spent little time together, as Goulston was due to rejoin his battalion in the first week in June. During the next three months, Jean was able to see Stan intermittently and she was present[21] in the enthusiastic crowd watching a parade of the battalion in Dubbo in September.

The battalion's existence on paper had been rapidly transformed into a real battalion of over nine hundred men[22] assembled for their training at Greta in New South Wales. It eventually contained 1,500 men from all walks of life. Some of the new battalion were raw recruits while others had had CMF experience. In its formation, Captain Goulston was among the five officers first appointed to support Lieutenant Colonel Macgillicuddy. The newly married Goulston duly arrived at Greta in the first week of June 1940. As Regimental Medical Officer, and its only doctor, he was responsible for establishing a medical facility, known in Army language as the Regimental Aid Post (RAP). An RAP is intended to function like a small emergency department in a modern hospital and has to be capable of treating ambulant patients as well as having hospital-type beds for the more seriously injured or ill. As we shall soon see, RAPs can be housed in a variety of physical structures, especially when in the battlefield. Goulston was also responsible for training his own staff for the RAP. These staff included stretcher-bearers/ medical orderlies (who were soldiers with the ability to play a musical instrument, recruited to serve also in the battalion band) and non-commissioned officers (NCOs) trained to administer first-aid and morphine injections at the battlefront.

His first RAP at Greta was in a converted mess hut. Supplies including beds, instruments, and drugs[23] were provided by the Red Cross and the Battalion's Comforts Fund.[24] One early task was to organise the vaccination of over one thousand men against smallpox, typhoid and tetanus – a task not without its dramas. As recorded by Goulston, the Regimental Sergeant Major volunteered to be the first vaccinated, to show the men that injections were not to be feared. Fronting up with his arm bared, the Sergeant Major's sighting of the needle saw him slide 'sweetly to the ground in a dead faint'.[25]

It was not long before Goulston's medical skills were tested, as in June and July the camp experienced major outbreaks of influenza, pharyngitis, tonsillitis and rubella. The influenza epidemic was the worst, for in one week, seventy-five of his men had to be admitted to the nearby 2nd/5th Army General Hospital (AGH) and during the two weeks of this epidemic, 325 men were treated by bed rest in the camp. Goulston and his partly trained medical orderlies also had to treat many beginner soldiers for sore and blistered feet brought about by long marches – a core element of fitness training.

In addition to being their doctor, Goulston was required to take part in all training activities including route marches and revolver practice.[26] Although young and inexperienced as a doctor, he was a quick learner. He soon could differentiate 'between sufferers and merely complainers' and found himself as a 'counsellor and advisor' to the men.[27]

In early September 1940, the battalion was relocated to a new camp near the New South Wales town of Dubbo. The residents of the town responded enthusiastically when the battalion conducted a formal march down the main street. Here, in distinction to Greta, there was no AGH or camp hospital and Goulston was now entirely responsible for the medical care of the battalion. The stay in Dubbo was brief, as within ten days, notice was received to prepare for embarkation abroad. At this point, the battalion had had four months of training. The battalion was granted seven days of pre-embarkation leave, from 20 to 27 September.[28] This was to be the last time that Stan would see Jean for two years. Unbeknown to Jean, before her husband departed Australia he made arrangements that she should receive roses from him every Friday evening during his absence.[29]

On 30 September, half of the battalion left Sydney on a Dutch ship, the HMAT SS *Johan de Witt*,[30] with most of the soldiers accommodated in 'converted holds'.[31] The other half went by train to Melbourne to board another converted Dutch ship, the HMAT SS *Niew Zealand*. The medical complement of the battalion included a dentist, a doctor (Goulston) and four nurses from the Australian Army Nursing Service. The two ships met in Melbourne and on the journey to the Middle East were escorted by HMAS *Perth* and later HMAS *Canberra*.

In a voyage that took five weeks (with brief stops at Colombo and Aden), the temporary hospital that the medical team set up on board their ship was not unduly busy. Dr Goulston saw only one case of typhoid fever and a man with epilepsy[32] but the ship did have one death, occasioned by accident when a young soldier fell down some steps at night and broke his neck. He was dead when found the next morning. There were five men who presented with broken bones and a few with sprains requiring his attention. On the voyage, Goulston was able to complete the training of his orderlies in first-aid, splinting and some other medical matters including treatment of men exposed to war gases.

The battalion disembarked at El Kantara, at the northern end of the Suez Canal, and were transferred by train to a new tented camp at Julis in Palestine, just a few miles north of Gaza (Palestine then being controlled by the British). Here Goulston established his RAP in a large tent with an adjacent second tent to serve as the battalion hospital, capable of accommodating ten patients. Conditions at first were difficult, as there was heavy rain and the area was badly drained. In the first two weeks, Goulston had two cases of meningitis and the camp had to be quarantined.[33] Other medical problems encountered were 'mild epidemics of enteritis' and sandfly fever.[34] By 11 November, the battalion was back in full training, now in a desert environment. The medical officer was expected to be as fit as his troops, so once again Goulston was doing pistol practice and joining the now 1,500 men on marches, carrying a pack on his back.[35]

One of Goulston's responsibilities as Regimental Medical Officer was to monitor not only the health of his battalion but also their fitness for battle. In his first report after arrival in Palestine, he declared that the long sea trip had rendered the troops 'soft'. This was probably a reflection of his and his orderlies' need to treat over one hundred men with foot complaints within ten days of renewing training at Julis. Some of the battalion's heavy equipment arrived in late November (but not the Bren guns, anti-tank weapons and signalling equipment they were anticipating) and included thirty small trucks, one of which was allocated to the RAP and became Goulston's mode of transport for the next eleven months.

The transport officer gave every truck a name, linked alphabetically to the battalion company (A, B, C and D) to which the truck was allocated. The officer must have had a wry sense of humour because the name he chose for Goulston's truck was 'ASPRO', which was emblazoned above the front windshield.[36] 'Aspro' was not to survive the war intact.

Soon after arriving in Palestine, concerns had arisen regarding the health of the battalion's Commanding Officer, Lieutenant Colonel Macgillicuddy. Goulston had been instructed by a 'very senior Army Officer' that he was to report to him should he find that the Commanding Officer was unfit to lead the battalion into action. On 26 December 1940, Macgillicuddy was so unwell that Goulston had him admitted to hospital. The nature of this illness is not recorded in the history of the 2nd/1st Pioneers[37] and its absence suggests that he may have had a mental breakdown. Young Dr Goulston did not shirk his onerous responsibility and, having assessed the patient carefully, advised his seniors that Macgillicuddy was unfit for work.[38] The Commanding Officer was relieved of his command and repatriated to Australia. This must have been a difficult and burdensome decision for Goulston, as it is one of the few aspects of his time in the Middle East of which his family remain acutely aware.[39]

On 29 December, the battalion was moved forward to another training camp near Alexandria in Egypt and here they experienced their first severe dust storm, a forerunner of what was to come in Libya. Their stay was brief, as on 19 January they were moved by ship and road to Salum and five days later were moved into Tobruk, the town having been taken from the Italians by the Allies two days earlier. The Pioneer Battalion history records that some of its soldiers celebrated this arrival at the front with a cache of cognac left behind by the routed Italians. More valuable for the Australians were many trucks abandoned by the Italians, as well as medical equipment of all kinds and a brand new microscope. Goulston kept the microscope with him throughout the war and for many years afterwards, but in 1970 he found an appropriate means of sending it back to Italy.[40] So Goulston was at the battlefront at Tobruk at the age of twenty-five, just nine months after being called up.

CHAPTER 4

A Rat of Tobruk

To appreciate why withstanding the siege of Tobruk was so important for the Allied Forces in World War II and to understand why Stanley Goulston quietly took more pride in being a 'Rat of Tobruk' than all of his other achievements, it is necessary first to take a step back and examine how the war had progressed from its declaration in September 1939.

World War II officially began when Hitler sent his German troops into Poland on 1 September 1939 and Britain and France made their responses clear two days later. Poland was quickly overrun and occupied. This success for the Germans was repeated in the next few months with the invasion and occupation of Norway and Denmark on 9 April 1940, followed by the invasion of Belgium, Luxembourg, Holland and most of France beginning on 10 May, the same day that the British Prime Minister, Neville Chamberlain, resigned and was replaced by Winston Churchill. German tanks and troops were so powerful and effective in their invasion of France[1] that they forced the Allied Army back to the French shores, necessitating the famous evacuation of 340,000 British and French soldiers off the beaches of Dunkirk in late May and early June 1940. While that evacuation was a remarkable success, allowing the Allies time and personnel to regroup, it was also a major defeat. One of its consequences was to make it much easier for the German planes, now located in Normandy, to bomb Britain.

Hitler planned to invade Britain and preceded this with intensive night-time bombing of London as well as other British cities. This phase of the war was known as the 'Battle of Britain' and lasted from July to September 1940. It was followed by the 'Blitz', the name given to further German bombing raids throughout Britain over the next twelve months aimed at disrupting manufacturing and military bases and airports. Hitler's invasion plans were deferred initially because of lack of airpower. Later, through events in Greece and in Libya triggered by the unpredictable behaviour of the fascist Italian dictator, Benito Mussolini, Hitler's invasion of Britain was put on hold indefinitely.

At the outbreak of the war, Mussolini declared that Italy would remain neutral. However, within months, encouraged by Hitler's successes and anticipating the invasion of Britain, Mussolini opportunistically decided to enter the war on Germany's side. With Hitler's encouragement, he first sent 250,000 troops into Libya, the aim being to attack the Allied Forces protecting Egypt, the Suez Canal and the British naval base at Alexandria.

However, Mussolini's Italian troops, including some of their leaders, did not share his desire for war. The planned confrontation of Mussolini's troops in Libya with the Allied Forces stationed at the border between Libya and Egypt was delayed many weeks by the commanding officer, who doubted the wisdom of his leader's order. Mussolini, desperate to impress Hitler, then ordered his troops to invade Greece, without first notifying Hitler. This invasion was a military disaster for the Italians as the Greeks readily repelled them. Concerned that his ally, Italy, not be defeated and concerned equally that the Axis Forces not lose momentum against the British forces, Hitler decided to send his own troops into Libya to confront the British and at the same time, send troops into Greece. These decisions led to the delay of an invasion of Britain. Later, Hitler's attack on Russia in June 1941 led to further deferment of any land assault on Britain.

Thus in early 1941, North Africa, particularly Libya and western Egypt, became the central battleground of World War II. It was here that Australian troops first encountered the German Army and with a significant impact. Germany was determined to maintain the upper hand and, if possible, take control of the Suez Canal out of the hands of the British. Loss of the canal would have severely impeded the contributions of men, arms and supplies from the British Empire nations of India, Australia and New Zealand; its defence was imperative. In addition, were the combined German and Italian forces to defeat the Allied Forces in North Africa, the war may have been lost, well before the USA decided to join the conflict.

This setting helps to explain how Tobruk came to be the focal point of the North Africa campaign for well over a year. Tobruk in peace-time was a small Libyan coastal town with a population of around 7,000 people, a mixture of Italian settlers and servicemen together with some Arabs. Tobruk is situated on the Mediterranean coast some 800 km from the capital Tripoli to the west and 300 km from the Egyptian border to the east. Apart from a small number of other coastal towns, this vast expanse of Libya that extends from Tripoli to the Egyptian border is desert. Access of Axis military forces from Tripoli towards Egypt was limited then to a coastal road that took in Tobruk and a second inland road that also passed through the town. Notably, Tobruk had a deep harbour – the only valuable Libyan harbour other than the one at Tripoli – and it had the additional attraction in a desert area of a reliable water supply.

Following the Italian Army's defeat of the Turks in 1912, Libya was effectively an Italian colony. Italian settlers made the small town of Tobruk attractive and self-sufficient. In addition, the Italian Army, recognising the strategic nature of the port, had turned Tobruk into a garrison, and maintained a strong army and navy presence. In the years leading up to World War II, the Italians had constructed a defensive perimeter line of approximately 45 km to protect the town from inland invaders.

For the Allied Forces to defeat the Axis powers in Libya, a key step was to take control of Tobruk. This was achieved when, on 21 and 22 January 1941, the Allies, advancing from Egypt, overthrew the Italians. The Allied Forces included the Australian 6th Division, which performed magnificently. This was the first occasion of action by any Australian force in this war. The battle was brief, lasting less than forty-eight hours, and resulted in taking 27,000 Italian soldiers as prisoners, the loss of life of forty-nine Allied servicemen and injury to another 306 men. The Allies also collected over 200 Italian trucks as well as arms, ammunition, medical supplies and food supplies.

Having gained control of Tobruk, the Allies pressed on west hoping to push the Italian Army back to Tripoli. However, by now Germany had sent its own force to bolster the Italians and a powerful force it was, led by General Erwin Rommel who had been very successful in the campaign in France. The Allied Forces were handicapped as, at this moment, Churchill insisted that the Australian 6th Division, now battle hardened, be moved to defend Greece, in what proved to be a military catastrophe. The 6th Division was replaced by the Australian 9th Division, which had been put together hastily and was not yet ready for such a difficult task, although later it performed admirably. The Allies were quickly pushed back to the fortress of Tobruk.

At this critical time, the British High Command and Prime Minister Churchill were deeply alarmed at the lack of resources to defend Cairo, Alexandria and the Suez Canal. They needed more time to get additional personnel and arms to Egypt. They realised that if the Germans took Tobruk, the Axis Forces would be able to receive supplies of fuel and arms from Tripoli by ship to Tobruk rather than by the much less efficient 800-km trip by road, making a successful advance to the Suez Canal more feasible. Thus then, and in hindsight, it was seen that the outcome of World War II hung on defending Tobruk against siege for long enough that the forces in Egypt might be massively strengthened. And this was a siege to be conducted by the best equipped and best led forces that Germany could assemble.

After the rapid retreat to Tobruk, there were too many soldiers and locals in the town to house and feed,[2] so a large number of Allied troops (but not including any Australians), as well as many Italian and Arab residents and Italian prisoners, were shipped to Egypt. This left a force of approximately 23,000 to defend Tobruk. This included 14,000 Australian soldiers (the 9th Division and the 2nd/1st Pioneer Battalion) as well as soldiers from Britain and India. Later a free Polish force came in to provide relief.

To accurately trace the history of Goulston's battalion, we need once more to briefly take a step back. On 24 January, two days after the 6th Division had contributed mightily to the taking of Tobruk, another Australian battalion, the 2nd/1st Pioneers, for which Dr Stan Goulston was the Regimental Medical Officer, moved into Tobruk. Goulston, who graduated from Sydney University Medical School at the beginning of 1939 and was young and inexperienced,[3] served as Regimental Medical Officer to the Pioneers for eight months during the siege of Tobruk. During this time, he won a Military Cross and was mentioned in dispatches twice.

Goulston has written and spoken about his experiences at Tobruk but these accounts have mainly focused on the nature of his medical responsibilities and on the facilities at his disposal. To know about the trials, deprivations and dangers that he and his comrades were exposed to, other accounts need to be consulted.[4] Leaving aside almost daily exposure to air-raids by the Germans and shelling by German and Italian artillery, there were other trials. In the desert, the days brought unbearable heat while the nights could be freezing cold. Flies, fleas and ticks were a continuing hazard.[5] Water supplies were restricted and the men had a ration of only one bottle per day for drinking, shaving and personal hygiene.[6] Severe dust storms (locally called the Khamsin and in Egypt, the Khamaseen) could arise suddenly and bring visibility down to a few metres. The fine dust permeated everywhere. The only benefit of the Khamsin was that the enemy was equally affected, such that hostilities ceased for the duration.

In his accounts, Goulston also omitted a dramatic event that took place as the battalion first entered Libya from Egypt. He told his family this story late in his life.[7] A group of nomadic Arabs approached his team for help. He saw that a woman in the group had a gangrenous leg, the result of an injury from an Italian Army booby trap. Her survival depended on urgent amputation. A barn served as an operating theatre, one of his staff gave the chloroform anaesthetic and he operated with a carpenter's saw that had been sterilised in boiling water. The woman made a full recovery.

At first, the work of the Pioneer Battalion at Tobruk was to repair the badly damaged port facilities and the bombed roads in and nearby the town and to help salvage equipment left by the Italian Army. The battalion's first casualties involved soldiers who encountered a mine while working to build a detour around a bombed bridge west of Tobruk. One soldier was killed and four were wounded. As the Allied Forces had decided to pursue the retreating Italians west to Benghazi, hoping to capture that city, the Pioneer Battalion soon found itself spread out on the road from Tobruk to Derma about 160 km west, and then further along this road to Benghazi, another 200 km west, still repairing roads and bridges. This work occupied them until the end of February. During this time, Goulston and his driver in 'Aspro' sought to visit these teams as often as possible to conduct 'sick parades'.[8]

It was at this point that the bulk of the Australian troops (the 6th Division) involved in the capture of Tobruk were withdrawn and sent to Greece. They were replaced by the 9th Division, a force less battle ready. At about the same time, well-armed German forces led by Rommel arrived by road from Tripoli to strengthen their Italian friends. The Australian and British advance towards Benghazi had to be abandoned and a retreat to Tobruk under very difficult circumstances was ordered on 3 April. Goulston in 'Aspro' was caught up in a mass of vehicles seeking the safety of Tobruk as quickly as possible. Most of the Allied Force made it back intact, although there were casualties and some prisoners were taken by the Germans. By 8 April, all members of the Pioneer Battalion were inside Tobruk; then began the long siege of the town.

Now the Pioneer Battalion soldiers were ordered to use their infantry skills and were allocated to defensive posts outside the township. To describe fully how Tobruk was defended would take up much of this book; instead readers who wish to know more may consult one or more of the histories written either soon after the events,[9] or later when information gleaned from German war records became available.[10] In the briefest of summaries, the Australian officer in charge of all Allied Forces at Tobruk (Australian, British, Indian and the later Polish brigade), General Leslie Morshead, chose to utilise existing Italian defensive structures built in two lines well beyond the township. The outer line, known as the Red Line, extended over a semi-circular perimeter of 28 miles (45 km) from the coast west of Tobruk to the coast east of the town. Spread out along this line were 137 underground concrete bunkers which provided protection for defenders as well as observation posts of the few incoming roads.[11] Additional defences – which the Allies soon sought to strengthen – were trenches, tank traps, mines and barbed-wire barriers. All hands were applied to this work, including those of the Australian officers. This resulted in one anecdote that must have spread rapidly through the Australian soldiers.

The story is recounted by Peter FitzSimons in his 2006 book, *Tobruk*. A neatly attired young British Army Captain sought to reprove a dusty Australian 'Digger' working on deepening a trench for not saluting an officer. The 'Digger' turned his back on the Captain, slowly put his shirt back on and turned around brushing the dust off his epaulettes that revealed he was a Major. He then explained to the Captain, in earthy language, that he was the Commanding Officer of these men and that they did not even salute him. He finished by telling the Captain, 'Now, as I outrank you, stand to attention and salute'.[12]

A key element of Morshead's approach to defence was to seek to keep the enemy under pressure with regular night-time raids – raids which also collected valuable intelligence and sometimes prisoners for interrogation. This approach meant that during the siege, even when there was no full onslaught by the Germans, every Regimental Aid Post (RAP) was always at readiness to receive injured soldiers. The defence posts were well dug in, but because the surrounding territory was mostly flat bare desert, it was unsafe to try to move injured or unwell soldiers from the Red Line in daylight hours. Those hours at the Red Line were for soldiers to attempt to rest. Those seeking medical help could only move to the RAP under the cover of dark.

Approximately two miles back, between the Red Line and the township, was a second line of defensive posts along what became known as the Blue Line. At different times in the coming months, troops of the Pioneer Battalion manned posts on one or other line. In his eight months at Tobruk, Goulston's battalion moved four times and as a result he established four RAPs. In his later description of the work in which he was engaged at Tobruk,[13] Goulston focused mainly on the fourth of these posts, probably because its physical structure was so unusual and possibly because this was the post at which he was based for the longest time.

In each case, Goulston was expected to establish an RAP in close proximity to his troops. His first RAP was a tent partially protected by overhanging rock and hopefully protected by a large Red Cross flag.[14] His second was in a wadi (a deep, dry water course) just behind Fort Pilastrino.[15] It was constructed of sandbags and a tarpaulin roof.[16] In a bombing and shelling raid which destroyed Fort Pilastrino and resulted in many casualties, Goulston had his first real taste of war. He was involved in caring for the injured while under attack and then urgently relocating his RAP staff and injured troops at 2 a.m. to a site that had been used for an earlier RAP.[17] This site consisted of three underground dugouts, each 10 ft by 12 ft,[18] and provided adequate safety for that rotation to the front. During the attack and in the task of relocation, Goulston remained calm and devoted his attention to the men under his care.[19]

In June, the battalion was back in action, now manning a section (posts S 11 to S 27) of the Red Line on the north-western perimeter. The battalion headquarters was a mile or so back in a wadi, behind one of the few landmarks in the area, a large old fig tree. This area became known as Fig Tree Hill. As a landmark, it was also a target for enemy shelling. Goulston found a safe place for his RAP, a large natural cave, concealed immediately below the fig tree.[20] In the immediate vicinity of the cave was an ancient Jewish burial ground and it was believed that the cave, too, had been used for burials. The cave consisted of three natural rooms, the largest of which measured 20 ft x 15 ft and had a ceiling height of 6 ft. This was used for medical examinations and also doubled as the sleeping quarters for Goulston and the battalion chaplain. The second 'room', which measured 16 ft x 16 ft but had a ceiling height of only 4 ft, was used as a sick bay and as sleeping quarters for the medical orderlies. Goulston estimated that the RAP could accommodate twenty-five or thirty wounded men.[21] The third 'room' was small but big enough to be used as a pantry and cookhouse. In daytime, sufficient natural light came from two air holes in the roof of the cave but at night, hurricane lamps were needed.[22] His RAP was of sufficient interest to attract a visit from the overall commander of the Tobruk forces, General Morshead, whom Goulston described as 'an excellent general' and 'a great gentleman'.[23]

While the occupants of the cave may have been safe, the troops on the Red Line were not. The Pioneer Battalion history records that from 6 June until 1 July, some 4,200 shells fell within 100 yards of the posts which the men were holding. During this rotation, Goulston and his driver, using 'Aspro' at night near the front line, strayed on to a mine.[24] The front end was badly damaged[25] and the truck could not be repaired. Fortunately Goulston was unharmed, but his driver suffered an injury that led to his being returned to Alexandria for treatment.[26]

The cave RAP was only three-quarters of a mile from the Red Line and was close to the Battalion Headquarters. It was not safe to bring an ambulance to the RAP, so four stretcher bearers were used to carry injured or sick soldiers needing hospital care a quarter of a mile to a wadi where the ambulance was concealed. Wherever possible, Goulston and his assistants were expected to manage less serious injuries and illnesses at the RAP. For example, in June the commonest problem treated was mild dysentery and most sufferers were able to return to their posts in two to three days.[27] Only soldiers with more serious illnesses and injuries were transported to the Australian 4th Army General Hospital (AGH), a 600-bed complex housed in variously protected buildings within Tobruk. One building was a concrete shelter next to the harbour, capable of housing seventy stretcher cases awaiting a moonless night for evacuation by ship to Alexandria.[28]

Goulston's RAP was linked by telephone line to Battalion Headquarters and to all the frontline battalion posts. At three of these posts, a forward RAP substation was established, staffed by an NCO, authorised to give morphine injections, and a medical orderly equipped with a first-aid kit. Sick or injured soldiers were brought back to the main RAP at night by the trucks that delivered a hot meal to the troops. Goulston's 'sick parade' hours were from 11 p.m. until 2 a.m.

Goulston sought to keep in personal contact with his troops. Despite the dangers of moving around in daylight because of the risk of sniper fire, he managed to visit at least one forward RAP each day. This took a lot of courage and must have been one of the many reasons that the battalion held him in high regard. He had earlier demonstrated his courage and calmness under pressure during the bombing raid and artillery barrage that forced the relocation of the RAP in the middle of the night at Fort Pilastrino. For this example of bravery and leadership, he was awarded the Military Cross.[29] The citation[30] for the award read:

> As R.M.O. of this Battalion, Capt. Goulston has set a splendid example of devotion to duty and courage under fire. At all times during the operations in Libya he has carried out his duties without regard to enemy action. On one occasion in the PILASTRINO SECTOR, the enemy heavily dive bombed our batteries positions in the vicinity of which was the R.A.P. Despite the attack and the fact that wounded men in the R.A.P. were effected [sic] by the proximity of the bombs, this Officer remained cool and carried on with his work and by his example held the men together until they could be evacuated. Although normally regarded as a non-combatant, Capt. Goulston set an inspiring example to every member of the Battalion.

The most that Goulston ever said about the incident leading to the award of the Military Cross was 'for quite a while we were under direct fire'.[31] For further bravery, he was twice mentioned in dispatches.[32] In the same months that Goulston was at Tobruk, another Australian doctor from the Royal Prince Alfred Hospital, Bill Morrow, was second-in-charge of the 2nd/5th AGH – a field hospital – and was in danger with the troops in Greece and in Crete where evacuations were needed. For his courage, calmness and leadership after his commanding officer was killed, Morrow was awarded a Distinguished Service Order (DSO).[33] As will be seen,

Morrow and Goulston (the latter, twelve years younger) were to have a very close professional relationship and parallel professional careers.

Another measure of the high regard in which Goulston was held by the troops was his award of a Rats of Tobruk medal. Before describing this award, it is necessary to explain the origin of the nickname, 'Rats of Tobruk'. At the beginning of the siege, the Germans were very confident of overwhelming the defences of Tobruk, so much so that leaflets were dropped recommending surrender. However, morale was high inside the garrison and these leaflets were treated with the disrespect that might be expected of Australian troops. At around the same time, the English-speaking German radio propaganda broadcaster, William Joyce, nicknamed 'Lord Haw-Haw', was nightly heard to depict the situation inside Tobruk as perilous and on one night was heard to say that the inhabitants were living like rats.[34] This was immediately adopted by those inhabitants as their own nickname, the 'Rats of Tobruk'. The epithet has ever stuck in Australia's proud military history.

A little while later, some Rats of Tobruk medals were struck within the camp by a member of the Pioneer Battalion, Leonard ('Lofty') Barlow.[35] The medals were made by hand out of metal derived from an Italian shell case, a damaged German tank and a crashed German bomber. Even the 'ribbon' from which hung the medal (depicting a 'rat rampant') was made of metal. Inscribed on each medal are the words 'Presented by Lord Haw-Haw to the Tobruk Rats 1941'. Individually made, each medal is different in minor ways from the next. Goulston posted his medal home for safe-keeping; later, when he learned that his father had sought publicity for his award, he was distressed, as this was not his wish.[36]

It is still unclear how many of these medals[37] were made. In the official history of the Pioneer Battalion, it is said that a complete list of recipients and the whereabouts of these medals is unavailable.[38] However, Stan Goulston's family has a list compiled by a Tom Osborn in 2012 suggesting thirteen recipients. When in 2011 the Rats of Tobruk exhibition at the Australian War Memorial had added to it a medal belonging to Major General J.J. Murray, the accompanying documentation noted that 'around twenty' had been made.[39] One recipient was Stan Goulston[40] and the medal remains in the possession of his family. Newspaper reports at the time that Goulston received it stated, probably incorrectly, that he received the medal because he did not lose a patient through illness during the seven months when his battalion was in Tobruk. This seems to be highly unlikely, as the medal was made and awarded well before such statistics were available. It is much more likely to reflect the soldiers' awareness of Goulston's courage under fire. The news of the award rated a mention in his old school's magazine and there it was assumed that it was for 'unselfish devotion to duty'.[41] Other recipients included General Blamey[42] and Major General Morshead. Goulston later stated that he was prouder of this medal than of his Military Cross.[43] Certainly its award tells us much about the admiration and respect that his battalion had for this young doctor.[44]

Goulston sent home some other treasured Tobruk souvenirs. One was a metal ashtray with an image of the map of Australia mounted on it. It was made from the propeller of a German aeroplane shot down by the antiaircraft platoon of his battalion and inscribed on its base are the words 'Presented to Cpt S Goulston, RMO, from the boys of number 5 platoon, 2/1 Aust Pioneer Battalion, AIF, Tobruk 1941'. He was also given six handsome, inscribed egg-cups made from the tails of Italian two-inch shells.[45]

Goulston's RAP team was responsible for more mundane but still critical tasks, including overseeing the construction of temporary latrines and enforcing the rules of hygiene and safe disposal of human waste. In this they were successful, as very few cases of dysentery were seen.[46] Indeed at the end of June 1941, Goulston reported to his superiors 'these measures for hygiene had resulted in less evacuations because of illness than under peace time conditions in earlier locations'. As noted in the battalion history, 'this was despite the debilitating conditions in the area and its effect on the men whose average age is greater than in an infantry battalion'.[47]

When the battalion was withdrawn to the Tobruk township for periods of rest, Goulston remained active in the care of his troops. For example, he instigated group trips to the coast for swimming, partly for the exercise but also because he sensed that this would help those soldiers with foot complaints.

Despite the workload and the testing environment, Goulston found time to write to Jean once a week. Most or all of the letters arrived, as Jean stored them carefully and her family still hold them. In his letters home, Goulston signed himself 'Scipio Africanus', because the historic figure Scipio was one of his heroes,[48] while he addressed Jean as 'Topsy', a nickname he had given her. All outgoing mail was censored to ensure that vital information would not be released should the mail fall into enemy hands. Goulston censored the mail of those who reported to him, while someone higher up censored his letters. Jean's return letters were treasured at the time but have not been saved. Also treasured were two pullovers that Jean had knitted.[49] The nights in the desert could be very cold.

The 2nd/1st Pioneer Battalion finally left Tobruk on the night of 17–18 September 1941. For the battalion, the siege had lasted six months,[50] although at first they were told that they needed to hold Tobruk for only two months. They had contributed to delaying the German Army and allowed ample time for the forces in Egypt to be greatly strengthened. While the Germans were not defeated in the battle for Tobruk, they had been held at bay by a much smaller but very determined force. This sent the reassuring message that the Germans were not invincible and gave the Allied Forces greater confidence for the difficult times ahead.

Goulston remembered the departure vividly, luxuriating with fresh egg sandwiches and hot cocoa followed by a deep sleep on the deck of a British destroyer as it scurried back to Alexandria.[51] The departure was part of the overall withdrawal of all Australian troops. Between 17 and 27 September, during a moonless period,[52] some 6,000 Australian troops (including 554 wounded) were evacuated on Royal Navy and Royal Australian Navy ships to Alexandria and, at the same time, 6,300 fresh British troops were brought in. Amazingly each ship was usually turned around in two hours.[53]

From Alexandria, the Pioneer Battalion moved back to Palestine, where the 9th Division together with the Pioneers were formally inspected by General Thomas Blamey on 6 October. Training for the Pioneer Battalion began again in earnest in November, now as part of the 7th Division. During this time, troops were rewarded with generous leave to visit places nearby. Goulston visited Luxor, Tel Aviv and Jerusalem; at Jerusalem he managed to take in a concert and purchase a large batch of sports uniforms for the battalion.[54] At Tel Aviv on the night of 26 November 1941, he attended a performance of classical music and dance mounted by the Palestine Orchestra in conjunction with the dancers of Gertrud Kraus. The annotations on his programme show that he enjoyed the evening and suggest that he was keen to write to Jean about it.[55] He also attended an advanced field hygiene course at the American University of Beirut.[56] In this relaxed interregnum, there was now time for sport involving inter-battalion matches of rugby union and hockey. Goulston was selected as a member of the Pioneer Battalion hockey team.[57] He managed a trip to Damascus, where he purchased a hand-made rug from a street seller; it later graced the floor of his study at home for many years.

While Goulston was in the Middle East, Japan entered the war with its bombing of Pearl Harbor. Singapore fell to the Japanese on 15 February 1942. Australian forces were brought back to help defend their own country. By 12 March, Goulston's battalion was boarding a large, US luxury tourist ship at Port Tewfik for their trip home to Australia. The ship had been rapidly converted to a troop carrier and renamed the USS *Westpoint.* It was manned by US Navy personnel. It was said to be a very fast ship that could outrun submarines and destroyers and thus, for the voyage to Australia, it had no sea or air protection. As a form of protection against submarine attack, it changed course every few miles, zig-zagging its way to the west coast of Australia. It arrived in Fremantle on 25 March but the troops were not disembarked until the ship reached Adelaide, on 30 March. Here each man was given one free telegram to tell family that they were now in Australia, but soldiers other than officers were forbidden to reveal their location.[58] On receiving her telegram from Stan, his wife Jean, who had not seen him for two years, took a train to Adelaide to be with him – but only for a few days.

So Captain Goulston was back in Australia safe and sound, wondering where he would next be sent. There were rumours that it might be to New Guinea (today's Papua New Guinea), which the Japanese were threatening. However, in August 1942 Goulston learnt that he was to be relieved of his duties with the Pioneer Battalion by a Dr Geoff Dynon and thus it was Dynon who later went to New Guinea with the battalion, which again performed admirably. Goulston was sent for some additional training and was then ready to begin the next chapter of his Army life.

As a young man, Goulston may not have dwelt on how close he must have come to death or injury or capture by the enemy. Although classed as non-combatants, and protected to some extent by the conventions of warfare, Australian doctors were subject to a significant mortality rate. In an analysis of the records of the 708 doctors who served in the Australian Armed Forces between 1939 and 1942, there were fifty-two deaths (7.3%).[59] Of these, fifteen were killed in action, twelve died of disease (some as prisoners of war), twelve drowned at sea,[60] seven were executed by the Japanese and six died in accidents including plane crashes.

Long after the war, Stan Goulston discovered that his elder brother Eric, a surgeon also serving in the Army, had without Stan's knowledge tried to arrange a swap such that he would replace Stan at Tobruk. Stan was upset at this news, because he would not have wanted to leave 'his' battalion. He thought that his brother just wanted to be 'closer to the action' (i.e., nearer to the front line).[61] This may not have been the case, as Eric Goulston saw plenty of action in Ethiopia and in Greece[62] and was a Lieutenant Colonel when discharged from the Army at the end of the war. Instead he may have been concerned for his younger brother's safety.

What did Goulston make of this amazing experience at Tobruk? In 1987 when Goulston was invited to give the annual address at a Jewish returned servicemen's Remembrance Day dinner in Melbourne,[63] he finished his talk by describing his memories of Tobruk. These were some of his words:

> One remembers only the good things – the high morale, the courage and companionship of the men and officers of

> the battalion, and the humour which overcame tedium and boredom, and the occasional excitement … At night under the stars we had exotic talks on the brave new world we would build after the war.

He went on to acknowledge all those who had served in two world wars and finished by quoting the following two poems:

> **By Rupert Brooke, 1914**
> Blow out, you bugles, over the rich Dead!
> There's none of these so lonely and poor of old
> But dying, has made us rarer gifts than gold
> These laid the world away; poured out the red
> Sweet wine of youth; gave up the years to be
> Of work and joy, and that unhoped serene
> That men call age; and those that would have been
> Their sons, they gave, their immortality.
>
> **By Laurence Binyon, 1914**
> They shall grow not old, as we that are left grow old,
> Age shall not weary them, nor the years condemn,
> At the going down of the sun and in the morning,
> We will remember them.[64]

Are there any criteria by which Goulston's performance as the Regimental Medical Officer to the 2nd/1st Pioneer Battalion should be assessed? We don't know what expectations were created at his induction training in 1941, but in 1943, well after Goulston had returned to Australia, Captain P. Braithwaite published a detailed description of the role of the Regimental Medical Officer.[65] As his article had the imprimatur of the Director General of the Army Medical Services, it presumably accurately reflects the official view of the Army's expectations. Braithwaite emphasised that the role was 'to keep the unit fit and up to strength' and to do this especially by dealing with preventable diseases through educating soldiers about hygiene and sanitation and making sure that high standards were maintained. He also emphasised the importance of maintaining good rapport with all officers and soldiers and of regularly visiting men on the front line. Doing so would help to maintain the morale of his men and the medical officer's own morale. One imagines that Goulston read Braithwaite's article with interest. If he did, he should have been pleased that, by these criteria, he had performed exceedingly well. His seniors must have recognised this, as soon he was to be given a promotion and greater responsibilities.

CHAPTER 5

Army Life after Tobruk

When Goulston's 2nd/1st Pioneer Battalion arrived back in Australia, it was bivouacked briefly at Sandy Bay, north of Adelaide, and was then moved to Ipswich in Queensland.[1] Goulston may have anticipated remaining with the battalion and being sent to New Guinea (today's Papua New Guinea), where the Japanese were threatening invasion.[2] He had been with the battalion for over two years and knew the men well. However, this was not to be; in August 1942, Goulston was informed that he would be replaced in his battalion and he was ordered to proceed to Duntroon, the Australian Army's officer training academy in Canberra.[3]

Here he undertook three months of advanced training in all aspects of military organisation and responsibilities. He was the only doctor among a group of thirty young men from every branch of the services.[4] Goulston thought that the content and teaching of the course was superb and contrasted this negatively with his 1940 induction training for Army doctors. Successful completion of the course led to participants having the right to put 'SC' (Staff Corps) after their name, thereby giving them increased status in their service. During this time, Jean was able to come and stay in Canberra with a married couple they knew, so she and Stan were reunited once more.[5]

Soon after the course, Goulston was promoted to Major and appointed Deputy Director of Medical Services in Darwin in the Northern Territory, where he served for fourteen months, including two Wet seasons. At the time of this appointment, invasion by the Japanese Army was anticipated and there were 25,000 Australian troops and many US Air Force personnel encamped along the recently macadamised road between Darwin and Katherine.[6] Goulston recalled that Darwin had been subject to twenty or more bombing raids and that the government chose not to tell the Australian people.[7] His duties now were mainly administrative. He oversaw two temporary 1,200-bed hospitals, one in Darwin and the other in Katherine, and travelled between the troop camps to inspect medical facilities and to support the battalion medical officers. He estimated that the geographical area under his medical supervision was greater than that of England.[8] For a young doctor, this was a remarkable promotion and reflected the high regard that the Army medical hierarchy had for his ability.

Early in 1944, he was granted leave to sit the examinations for membership of the Royal Australasian College of Physicians (RACP), which were held in Sydney in April of that year. He passed at his first attempt and was now entitled to the post-nominal of MRACP (Membership of the RACP). That he found time and the energy to study for the written examination is remarkable in itself. That he passed the clinical examination with only fifteen months of hospital experience, now three years in the past, is even more remarkable.

In May 1944, his Commanding Officer informed him that he was to report immediately to the Army Headquarters in Melbourne. The Commanding Officer was unable to tell him why, as he himself did not know. In Melbourne, Goulston was told that he had a new job and within days he was on a troop ship on his way to London. He had been appointed to the role of Deputy Director of General Medical Services on the Australian Army Staff,[9] and in London he served as the Medical Liaison Officer for the Australian Army Medical Service from June 1944 until many months after the end of the war. Within a few months, the man he reported to retired, so he had full responsibility from then on. Goulston described his liaison officer duties in a paper published in the *Medical Journal of Australia* in 1947.[10]

To get to London safely, he travelled on a US military vessel, *Mariposa*, across the Pacific Ocean and through the Panama Canal to Boston. He took a train to New York and forty-eight hours later was on the RMS *Queen Elizabeth* with 18,000 US troops.[11] The liner zig-zagged across the Atlantic and in six days Goulston landed in Scotland. From there, he went by train to London via Newcastle, where he saw wounded soldiers arriving from the 'second front'.[12] He arrived in London on the day that Germany began firing V1 rockets on London. On 30 June 1944, one of those rockets landed near Australia House with the loss of over one hundred lives and many more people seriously injured. Although Goulston never spoke of this event, a fellow Australian officer John Buckley recalled that Goulston was rapidly on site to assist the wounded. Buckley observed that Goulston 'gave wonderful service to the wounded that day and after'.[13]

Major Goulston's new job was to pass on medical knowledge and news from Australia and to receive medical news and knowledge from the British and other forces to be relayed to Australia. The Allied Forces included military from several countries of what was then the British Empire – including Australia, New Zealand, India, Canada and South Africa. As these forces were fighting war in deserts, in jungles and in the air and at sea, it was seen by the medical arm of the military that the rapid sharing of medical information between the various forces was essential to the successful prosecution of the war.[14] The central hub where the medical information was being shared was London, which was moreover at that time the key city of the British Empire where most medical research was undertaken. Goulston was at the centre of all that was happening medically and was meeting senior people, including senior military medical officers as well as civilian leaders of medicine and medical research in the UK. Very heady days indeed.

An example of the medical breakthroughs that were being made during World War II included Australian research that led to effective prevention of malaria in its troops in tropical zones, so that its control 'became a powerful weapon'.[15] Another was British research that 'resulted in the total disappearance of typhus fever from British, Canadian and American troops in Europe'.[16] And it was in wartime that penicillin was developed and first used.[17] Furthermore, advances were constantly being made in methods of retrieving injured servicemen and in the management of those injuries and the management of shock.

A sadder example of Goulston's experience was an instruction received from Australia to find out more about the equipment and training of medical officers who were being parachuted with their battalions behind enemy lines. Goulston spent time at a secret location, studying their systems and getting to know these brave men. Back in London, he learnt that the men he had got to know were dropped into Germany shortly after his visit and were ambushed on arrival. Over half of the men were killed. Somebody had given away secret information.[18]

In London, Goulston stepped into a well-oiled system, the breadth and depth of which he described in his 1947 paper. The centre of the system was the office of the UK Director General of Army Medical Services (DGAMS) at the War Office.[19] The DGAMS oversaw a complex linkage of access to expertise. The Director General had senior advisers in medicine, surgery, pathology and hygiene and additional experts representing the best 'medical brains'[20] in the country. There was also a range of expert committees established through the Medical Research Council which were asked to report on specific emerging issues, such as jaundice and malaria in soldiers.

To assist information sharing, the UK Director General held monthly conferences in 'a concrete building under Whitehall',[21] attended by all his key people as well as representatives of the Navy and Air Force and relevant Ministries. Also invited were representatives of the medical services of all the Allied countries and the USA. Australia's Army Medical Service representatives were drawn from the office of the Australian Army based in London. To ensure appropriate medical representation at such conferences, from 1940, the Director General of the Australian Army Medical Service established the post of Medical Liaison Officer in London – the position to which Goulston was sent in 1944. The other Allied countries made similar appointments.

Goulston described his role as being 'the eyes and ears of his [Australia-based] Director General of Medical Services, keeping him in touch with trends of development in those fields of medical science which have a bearing on war'.[22] He was also the official spokesperson in London representing his Director General back in Australia. Goulston was at pains to point out that unless specifically asked, any opinion that he expressed was the opinion of his superiors and not his own. He described how important it was that the liaison officer should not be office bound but should make personal contact wherever possible when passing on information or seeking information. This practice must have greatly enhanced the number of valuable contacts that he made.

In his role, he attended the monthly conference already mentioned. He was free to sit in on various expert committees established by the Medical Research Council. He was expected to keep in contact with the UK Ministries of Health and of Supply, as his role also included helping to ensure that orders for medical and related supplies for the Australian Army were processed promptly. He was encouraged to attend medical society lectures and visit teaching hospitals when time allowed and to visit research centres and medical schools. He sent reports to the Director General in Australia each fortnight and sent cables for more urgent matters. In March 1945, he was sent to visit medical teams accompanying the British Army in eastern France as the Allies began their assault on Germany.

It was fortunate that he was stationed in London, as it enabled him to attend one of the ceremonies held every six months when military and civil awards were presented by the King – George VI in this case. Thus on 10 October 1944, he experienced the King pinning his Military Cross on his lapel.[23] This was well before his wife joined him, so the only family witness was a cousin, Myrtle Pinkus.

There is no diary of his activities, but from his 1947 published paper we know that he regularly attended meetings of the expert committees of the Medical Research Council and the monthly meetings of the Royal Society of Medicine – meetings that were closed and devoted to military medicine. He was a regular visitor to the British (later Royal) Postgraduate

Medical School at Hammersmith as well as to the Wellcome Research Foundation, the Imperial Chemical Industries Biological Research Centre in Manchester and the Schools of Tropical Medicine in London and Liverpool. When senior military medical men visited from Australia, it was Goulston's job to accompany them on all their official duties. As one example, he looked after Brigadier Neil Hamilton Fairley from Australia when he visited to brief the medical teams in London on the progress being made in malaria research at the Land Headquarters Medical Research Unit in Cairns.[24] It was at Hammersmith where he got to know several senior physicians, including Sir Francis Avery-Jones, Professor G.W. Pickering, Dr (later Professor) John McMichael and Dr Sheila Sherlock. When the war was over, he gained a training post under Dr Sherlock.

Given that Goulston was young and inexperienced medically, this was a wonderful learning environment into which he was thrust. That he made a positive impression on the senior medical people (both British and Australian) with whom he was dealing was borne out soon after the war had ended, when he applied for appointment as an Honorary Assistant Physician to his alma mater, the Royal Prince Alfred Hospital. Medical officers who provided strong references for him included Colonel John H. Anderson,[25] who among other things wrote: 'his work in London has brought him in frequent contact with many of the leaders of British Medicine and he was liked and trusted by them both for his personal qualities and his professional judgment'; Dr John McMichael,[26] Acting Director of the British Postgraduate Medical School, who wrote: 'I quickly came to form a high opinion of his capacity and was delighted when he expressed his intention of spending some time at the school on the cessation of hostilities'; and Brigadier Neil Hamilton Fairley,[27] who wrote: 'I was most impressed with his personality and his quite outstanding achievements as an administrator and medical liaison officer'.

During these busy first eighteen months in London, Goulston sat for and passed the examination for Membership of the Royal College of Physicians of London at his first attempt, without any recent involvement in civilian medical care. His superior, Colonel Anderson, commented later that this was 'specially meritorious as any preparatory work had to be done in his scanty off duty hours'. His having obtained this qualification was probably essential for the plan he had formulated for when the war was over.

The European phase of the war ended on 8 May 1945, although the Pacific phase still had a while to run. Goulston was in London to share the joy and excitement of Londoners when this was announced. More importantly, it was now feasible for Jean to join him and this she did, travelling alone on a troop carrier, arriving at Southampton within a few weeks, from where she made her way to London to meet her husband. Stan was not able to take even a short period of leave to welcome her at the docks.

Jean had experienced a difficult time during the war, feeling restless and unsettled. Work was now available for women and she was employed initially in Melbourne by the Vacuum Oil Company. Here she enjoyed a 'good boss'; her task was to log the fuel lorries, their loads and the distances driven. She moved to Sydney where she worked for a time in the stocks and shares division of the Bank of New South Wales. Still restless, she returned to Melbourne to see out the war years. Meeting Stan in London was later recalled as 'wonderful' and 'a great thrill'.[28]

The cessation of hostilities in Europe did not end Goulston's liaison work but his role did change. He was now overseeing and arranging the medical care of Australian troops who had been prisoners of war in Germany. He also found himself advising and directing fellow Army medical officers who, like him, were contemplating postgraduate training in civilian medicine in the UK before returning to Australia. By now Goulston knew many senior medical people in London, several of whom were also serving in the Armed Forces. Through these contacts, he helped several Australian doctors to find positions in Britain. He enjoyed this aspect of his work and was so impressed with the potential benefits of this role that he later recommended that a civilian counterpart office should be established in London.[29]

Earlier he had decided that, being in London, he should grasp the opportunity to obtain some postgraduate medical experience in London hospitals once war was over. One of the senior people he got to know was Dr John McMichael, who during the war was the Acting Director of the Postgraduate Medical School at Hammersmith.[30] McMichael had offered to help Goulston obtain a training post at the end of the war, and this he did. Goulston was given twelve months' leave from the Army, commencing in May 1946. Official leave was vital, as at the end of his clinical year he was able to go back into uniform and be repatriated at the Army's expense.

He applied for appointment to a highly sought-after post of Senior Medical Registrar at the Postgraduate Medical School at Hammersmith and won the position over well-qualified local applicants. He chose to work under Dr Sheila Sherlock. Goulston had met Sherlock several times during 1945 when he visited Hammersmith, as he was 'a frequent visitor on staff rounds'.[31] Dr Sherlock then was relatively unknown and was junior herself. She was three years younger than Goulston and had graduated top of her class in Edinburgh in 1941. Her appointment as Senior Lecturer to the Postgraduate Medical School was her first academic posting. She chose to specialise in liver disease and Goulston observed that she was applying serial use of the new technique of liver biopsy to follow the course of the illness of hepatitis. She subsequently was appointed Professor of Medicine at the Royal Free Hospital in London and became known and respected worldwide as a hepatologist (liver specialist), eventually as Dame Sheila Sherlock (1918–2001). Many Australian physicians later sought to train under her but Goulston was the first. They remained lifelong friends.

Goulston's position with Sherlock was unpaid but this was not a problem for him. It was the Army's practice to make all servicemen securely bank a proportion of their pay during the war (and for a married man, a fixed proportion also went directly to his wife). As a result, Goulston had accumulated around £4,000 – more than enough for him and his wife to live comfortably on for a year or so. He later described this year as 'the most wonderful year' and as 'a fantastic year', made more so by the birth of their first child, a girl they named Diana, in September 1946.

Diana's arrival was not without a funny anecdote. When Jean came into labour, Stan took her to the Hammersmith Hospital by bus. As was usual at that time, he was dismissed immediately and sent home with his wife's clothes bundled in his arms. It was now after midnight and he waited a long time for the two buses he needed. He was stopped twice by the police, since he looked to them like a thief. The second time, the policeman took pity on him and drove him home. About three hours later, he was woken by the hospital to say that the baby had arrived and he could now visit. Aware that he had lost six years of married life to the Army, Stan always saw Diana as a 'special gift'.[32]

While his remaining time in London was happy and memorable, there were difficulties. The 1946 winter was the coldest London had had for fifty years. They were able to rent a small, two-room flat in Marlborough Place, St John's Wood. The flat, like many London buildings, had been shaken by bombing, resulting in spaces around windows that let ice inside. They had a small fireplace but coal was rationed, so keeping the flat warm was difficult. Food was still in short supply and was rationed also. Despite these hardships, there was much that they enjoyed in London, such as concerts at Albert Hall. They were impressed by the spirit and comradeship of Londoners who had kept their entertainment venues open throughout the war. They went to Paris for a short break while cousin Myrtle cared for Diana. There they found things little different, as Paris was freezing and food was also limited.

Goulston's work with Dr Sherlock began in July 1946. While in London, he also spent three months at the London Children's Hospital, again in an unpaid post. During his time with Sherlock he was supervising House Officers (Resident Medical Officers, as they were then known in Australia). He quickly won Sherlock's confidence as she wrote in a reference in August that year: 'he has proved a very popular and lucid teacher in the Wards and during the past month has been in clinical charge of medical beds. He has a high sense of responsibility to his patients and an excellent clinical acumen.' Goulston found the work stimulating, as he felt that the hospital was at the forefront of advances in medicine. The technique of percutaneous liver biopsy had only recently been introduced[33] and

Sherlock's unit were using this monthly in selected patients to follow the course of hepatitis.[34] He was already interested in clinical research and during his stay commenced research into a means of prolonging the action of penicillin.[35]

While six months may seem a short period of training by modern standards, in those days postgraduate training was much briefer. In addition, there were few investigative techniques in gastroenterology to master other than liver biopsy, and high patient loads in London hospitals meant a rapid exposure to all the common illnesses. Goulston had not lived in his home city of Sydney since 1940 and had been out of Australia for much of the war. It was time to come home. He and his wife and baby Diana left Britain on the recently refitted RMS *Orion* on 25 February 1947,[36] Goulston in uniform and Jean as a fare-paying civilian. Jean was now in the early stage of her second pregnancy and was caring for baby Diana.

The family of three disembarked on 31 March 1947 and slipped quietly back into Sydney life. For the first three months, they lived with Stan's parents. Goulston wished to put his war experiences behind him and get back to the practice of medicine. For many years he ignored Anzac Day and made no effort to connect with his battalion comrades. His military exploits have not been forgotten by the Australian Jewish community. He is one of only four individual Jewish Australian servicemen mentioned on a website dedicated to maintaining the memory of the Holocaust.[37]

CHAPTER 6

Returning to Family Life

Elements of Stan Goulston's upbringing were not ideal, notably the authoritarian strictness and detachment of his father and the absence of his birth mother. Jean Danglow's childhood was somewhat different. She was the middle child of a rabbi whose approach to parenting had some similarities with that of Stan's father. Rabbi Jacob Danglow almost never went on holidays with his wife May and the children. He expected his children to attend the synagogue each week and to be well dressed when they did.[1] He was described as being 'engrossed in his congregation and with studying' and did not play with his children.[2] For Jean, this was counter-balanced by a warm and loving mother who was very much in charge of the non-religious decisions of the family. In passing, it should be noted that Stan and Jean made no criticisms of their respective fathers. They saw this male approach to parenting as unremarkable in an era when a wife stayed at home as the 'home-maker'.[3]

May Danglow (née Baruch) was indeed a talented and capable home-maker,[4] who loved to read to her children, entertain visitors, knit whenever she could, make jam when fruits were in season and preserve eggs.[5] She gave much time to her children[6] yet was still able to contribute her services to her husband's synagogue. Her home was a place where people in need were welcome. And we have seen how she supported her brother-in-law when he experienced a nervous breakdown during the Great Depression, and the manner in which, at very short notice, she made all the arrangements for Jean and Stan's wedding in 1940.

May's Australian mother, Bertha Michaelis, married Dalbert Baruch in Hamburg, Germany, where May and her brother Ernest were born. When Bertha was widowed quite young, she brought twelve-year-old May and May's brother back to live in her original family home, 'Linden', in Melbourne. Later, Bertha accompanied her daughter and son-in-law on a visit to Europe in 1913–1914 and through the vagaries of itineraries and transport, Bertha spent the entire World War I years in Britain.[7]

Jean recalled Stan's father, John Goulston, warmly. As a friend of Jean's father and later also the husband of her father's sister, Golda, John was a frequent visitor at the Danglow home when Jean was a child. He was known to the children as 'Uncle Jack' and was loved because he always had lollies in his pockets for them and because he played games with them. If Stan had been aware of these practices of his father when he himself was a boy, he would have had reason to be surprised.

Jean also recalled shopping excursions to Buckley and Nunn's department store and to Cann's store in the city.[8] These excursions included mother, grandmother and the three children and were made in the Rolls Royce owned by her grandmother's family, the Michaelises. Much to Jean's discomfort but to the delight of elder sister, Claire, the staff at Buckley and Nunn's used to 'bow and scrape' to the group.[9]

As children, Jean's and her sister's dresses were made by a dress-maker, Mrs Beckstrom, who came to their home. For women and girls, 'off the rack' dresses were not yet extensively marketed. Every winter until they were teenagers, the sisters received new velvet dresses, made to the same pattern but in a bigger size each year. Claire's was always brown velvet while Jean's was red. Jean's clothes and their colours were chosen by her mother up until the time when Jean became engaged to Stan. Everything in Jean's trousseau was hand-made by a German refugee who also came to the family home.

Her younger brother, Frank, was deeply religious and Jean seemed to have little difficulty accepting her father's strict religious regime. Her elder sibling, Claire, was different, chafing at restraints successfully[10] and determined to make her own way in life.[11] Claire became irreligious. Despite these differences, each girl served as a Prefect at Melbourne Girls Grammar School. Jean attended the University of Melbourne and completed a Bachelor of Arts degree, majoring in history. Claire had preceded her at the university, where she undertook the same degree.

As well as having a different disposition to her elder sister, Jean was handled differently by her parents. Claire insisted on having her hair cut short but Jean was compelled to keep her hair long and to wear plaits until she left school. Claire was three years older than Jean yet included her in all the various social activities of her university friends. They remained firm friends all their lives.

These then were the family backgrounds that Jean and Stan brought to their married life – a life that only truly began six years after their wedding in Melbourne in 1940. On arriving back in Sydney with baby Diana, they stayed with Stan's parents at Birriga Road in Bellevue Hill for three difficult months.[12] They were keen to live independently and soon found a small house to rent at 2 Chisholm Street in Greenwich. Here Stan set about creating a garden but in his efforts to dig out an Egyptian cassia bush he struck a water main and urgent help was needed.[13]

It was not long before Stan found a house to buy at 20 Shirley Road, Wollstonecraft. It was a two-bedroom house with an enclosed back verandah which had the potential to serve as an extra bedroom. Stan's father and Stan's brother Eric assisted Stan and Jean financially with this purchase.[14] Stan organised the move to Shirley Road while Jean was in hospital for the birth of their second child, Wendy. The couple also managed to buy a small, two-seater car – one that did not impress the older physicians at the Royal Prince Alfred Hospital, who deemed it unsuitable for one of their honorary physician colleagues.[15]

In 1949, the enclosed back verandah came into use with the arrival of third daughter, Sue. For a time, Jean was looking after three girls under the age of three – Diana, Wendy and Sue. Diana, the eldest, was adventurous while second child, Wendy, was not a good sleeper; her parents had to use the remedy of driving her around in their car to get her to sleep. Fourth daughter Sadhana (Anne) was born in 1952. The family was to live at Shirley Road for ten years.

As their first family home, Shirley Road remained Stan's favourite. The children also remember it well. Their father was home sufficiently to play with them often and to read to them. Their Uncle Eric, Aunt Nance and their cousins, Kerry and Jenny, lived in the same street. Sue and Wendy recall going to Uncle Eric's home as children on Friday nights and watching the dance hall opposite. Under the dance hall was the pre-school which the girls had attended. At Shirley Road, they had good neighbours who warmly welcomed the girls. On one side was Mr Norris who made toys for the girls, including go-carts and a board game. On the other side was Mrs Wilson, whom the girls called 'Wooshie', who acted as a dearly loved proxy grandmother to them all throughout their childhoods.[16] Their garden had a large peach tree and room for a swing and a cubby house in a tree. There was also room for Stan's passion for gardening and here he grew his first roses for Jean as well as azaleas and sweet peas, along with a range of vegetables.

As the girls grew, eventually it was clear that they needed a larger house and in 1957 one was purchased at 10A Gillies Street in Wollstonecraft. The house was to serve them well, as Stan and Jean remained there for over twenty-five years. It was an older home with five bedrooms, although some were small. The kitchen required complete renovation, as did the upstairs bathroom. There was a large backyard with a lawn tennis court that had had no attention for years. The surrounding fence was in disrepair. Left behind by a previous owner were an old roller and tennis net. Stan had visions of fixing the fence himself but soon found that the task needed a professional. However, he set to restoring the lawn surface, mowing it and rolling it regularly, and within a year it was ready for use. There was not a lot of space beyond the baselines but the surface was firm. Upkeep involved much work and when the girls were old enough they were expected to help with rolling, line-marking and pulling out paspalum grass on Sunday mornings.

Tennis then played a big part in the Goulstons' social life. Medical friends came regularly on Sundays to play and to enjoy a beer afterwards. Jean was also a keen tennis player and she had a regular group of ladies to play during the week. Stan made time for the upkeep of the court, which included renewing the white lines each week. If it rained, the lines were washed away. In 1958, Stan's younger brother, Roy, and his French wife, Simone, bought the house next door. Roy, too, joined in for tennis but was observed by his nieces to look out the window of his house each Sunday so that he could time his appearance for when all the preparatory work on the court had been completed.

As the daughters grew, two of them became keen players and had friends over for tennis. The tennis court served another purpose as well, as the Goulstons made it available on one occasion for the wedding of a Danglow relative; the court accommodated a large marquee.

At 10A Gillies Street there was a lovely front garden with an enormous jacaranda tree and nearby two macadamia nut trees. While the girls were young, the front garden was used for 'picnic' lunches, shared with their cousins next door. Stan also drove the family to the country for picnics, choosing spots adjacent to cow paddocks as part of his plan to teach his daughters to rejoice in nature.[17]

Adjacent to the tennis court there was space for a garden and Stan soon had flowers and vegetables growing. Along the front entrance path he planted roses, Jean's favourite flower, and he took great pride in them.[18] Their home was always 'full of flowers' and flowers were frequently given away as gifts.[19] Stan grew tomatoes, beans, potatoes, onions, carrots, silverbeet, broccoli and rhubarb. Gardening was a form of relaxation from work for him. Any spare time at weekends was spent in his garden. On weekdays, he would usually walk through to inspect and pull out a weed or two. His love of gardening came from the refreshing contrast he felt between his professional life of using 'mind, thought, opinion' and his need to have 'one's hands in soil and manure'.[20] Diana's hens, bantams and duck had their spot in the backyard. At both homes, the girls had a range of indoor and outdoor pets – lovebirds, goldfish in a tank, a dog and a cat and kittens.

Friday night at 10A was special, as it was family night when the extended family came together for Shabbat dinner. Roy and Simone and their four children came regularly from next door and grandfather John Goulston was a constant guest. Candles were lit and prayers were said before and after the meal.[21] These were evenings when the men did most of the talking. When his father was present, Stan would play dominoes with him after dinner.

The daughters as young girls fondly recalled visits from both grandfathers, whom they called respectively Grandpa (Goulston) and Papa (Danglow). Grandpa was perceived by the girls to be somewhat intimidating. Papa, who lived in Melbourne, visited less often. He willingly joined his granddaughters' games, told them children's stories from the Old Testament and sketched sunsets in their autograph books.

The four girls first attended the Lady Hayes pre-school and then the North Sydney Demonstration Primary School,[22] but as each girl finished Grade 2 she was moved to Presbyterian Ladies' College Pymble,[23] where all four completed their secondary education. This required a long walk to the train and a trip of ten stations. Two of the daughters thrived at the school. Later in life, Stan regretted that he had been unaware that one daughter really disliked her school experience.

As the children grew and as their father became much busier in his professional life, the pattern of daily activities gradually changed. The daughters were seeing less of their father and time spent with him became more precious. Stan took only two weeks off every summer for holidays and these were spent with his family, initially at a different beach resort each year, eventually settling on Mollymook where Jean bought a block of land and built a holiday house. For these holiday two weeks, Stan was relaxed with his children, swimming and fishing with them and playing Scrabble together. The garden at Mollymook also became a major focus for Stan.

For the May school holidays, the girls would go away for a week just with their mother and stay in a rented house. Stan would drive the family to the chosen place and collect them at the end of the week. When they were old enough, the September school holidays regularly included a week of downhill skiing. Jean had skied as teenager and a Sydney cousin was a keen skier, so the family group would be driven by the cousin to Thredbo where he had a membership of the Sydney Ski Club. Stan never tried to learn to ski.

When the girls were very young, there were weekend trips to the safe end of Balmoral beach. Later there were visits to Manly or Freshwater for the surf, where their father and Uncle Roy might body surf. Grandpa Goulston would take them to Manly, where they rode Shetland ponies but were not permitted to swim. These trips were remembered because their grandfather always wore a suit and had a woman driver named Dulcie who chain-smoked.

Stan's daughters warmly recall that, when they were very young, their father would often arrive home with chocolate frogs in his trouser pockets. He called the chocolates 'bees' and he would jump around causing the 'bees' to fly out of the pockets. The entire family had a passion for chocolates.[24] On Friday evenings, Stan would stop at his favourite shop, De Luca's, in the city and choose fresh fruit for his wife and daughters. At other times he would take them to De Luca's for their renowned fruit salad and ice-cream.

Other patterns of family life were affected by Stan's commitment to his work and Jean's firm support of this. At breakfast the children were clear that they were not to talk to their father while he was reading the paper, nor in the evening until he had eaten dinner. On weekdays in the evenings, the girls would have their dinner with their mother at 6 p.m. Stan usually arrived home at around 7.30 p.m. He would visit each child doing their homework, acknowledge them with a kiss or warm clasp of the shoulders and then join Jean for a drink (she, brandy and he, whisky) before eating his dinner separately. He would often give his young daughters a taste of his deliciously seasoned steak. After dinner he would retire to his study to read journals, prepare talks and, in the early years, smoke a pipe. Again the house was kept quiet so as not to disturb their father; this was not usually a problem as the girls were committed to their own homework. If any daughter needed help with their homework, their father was available.[25] Sometimes he surprised a daughter with a relaxed attitude to homework.[26]

Often one or other of the girls accompanied their father on a Saturday morning on hospital rounds and would read a book in the car while he visited his patients. Otherwise a common Saturday routine was for the girls to accompany their mother to the North Shore Synagogue and come home to a roast meal that Jean had prepared.

Growing up, the girls were all keen readers and also enjoyed listening to the radio and to music.[27] Jean would often have classical music playing while the family ate their meals and while she knitted awaiting her husband. Jean made sure that her daughters were introduced to classical music by taking each in turn to concerts in Sydney Town Hall. The two elder girls learnt to play musical instruments; the third daughter was 'scheduled' to learn the cello but this never eventuated. When television arrived in their home in 1960, they were permitted to view it but with strict limits. The girls participated in various sports at school including tennis, basketball, hockey and swimming. Their mother regularly came to watch, but 'Dad was always working'.[28]

With her husband deeply involved in his profession and the girls becoming more independent, Jean pursued her own artistic, sporting, philanthropic and other interests. Her father had introduced her to tennis and golf and she played each sport at a high level. She joined the Monash Golf Club[29] and played regularly. She had learned to ride horses as a child and she enjoyed this when living in Melbourne before she married. She was interested in horse racing and would occasionally have a bet. She loved to read and to knit; her mother, a keen knitter, had taught her this skill when Jean was a young child. Jean spun her own wool. She was never idle. She took up pottery, bridge, print-making, etching and cake decorating. In her eighties, her eyesight no longer quite up to tennis, she took up lawn bowls.

Of these activities, the one that she was most dedicated to was pottery. She took this up in 1965 and became a serious and accomplished potter and an exhibiting member of the Potter's Society. She studied the work of others at home and when travelling abroad, in Japan and the UK. She became friends with leading Australian potters, including Jean Higgs.[30] She had her own studio at home, with a potter's wheel and two kilns. She exhibited her work in several shows. Her daughters are the proud possessors of some beautiful examples of her work. Many friends received pottery as gifts.[31]

Jean Goulston was active in the North Shore Synagogue and served as a volunteer for charities that were raising funds for the Friends of the Hebrew University and for the University of Sydney. She was a volunteer for Meals on Wheels for thirty years. She was known in the community for her friendliness, wise advice, generosity and willingness to assist those in need.[32] Her service to the community and her standing in the Australian Jewish community led to a detailed description of her career appearing in a 1987 book about Jewish women in the history of New South Wales.[33]

Jean was always polite, calm, patient and even-tempered.[34] Some spoke of her serenity and one daughter observed that her mother seemed to have taught herself a form of relaxation or meditation. To people she had not yet got to know, Jean appeared reserved. Those who knew her were struck by the warmth apparent in her brown eyes.[35] She never swore; her daughters recalled that the worst words she ever used were 'dirty dog', 'Oh Lord' or 'a nasty piece of work'. She was reluctant to give advice unless asked. Although less religious than her father, she remained close to him.

She was a warm, generous host who liked to cook – one specialty was chocolate mousse – and as will be seen, she was given many opportunities to entertain her husband's professional visitors to Sydney. She was also a good listener at dinner parties, preferring not to speak about herself. On such occasions, the four daughters would assist their parents as 'hostesses'. One daughter recalled that the highlight for her was to finish off any leftovers of their mother's delicious chocolate mousse or zabaglione. After the guests had departed, the girls would help with the dishes while Stan sought their feedback as to how the evening had gone.

Each Passover, until it became too much for them, Stan and Jean hosted Seder night dinner at their home. Seder is the ceremony performed in association with a special meal on the first evening of Passover. Through prayers and songs, the departure from Egypt over 3,000 years ago is commemorated. These were large gatherings of the extended family and there could be up to twenty-five members present. The traditional Seder meal and order of readings were carefully maintained by Stan. He was interested in good wines and subscribed to the Wine Society, so dinner guests were well provided for.

Although Jean and Stan adhered less formally to Jewish religious practices than their parents, they did not ignore this aspect of the girls' upbringing. The children were obliged to attend the North Shore Synagogue with their mother and would accompany their father and mother to the Great Synagogue when their father was free of medical rounds on the Sabbath or for important days such as Yom Kippur.[36] All four girls prepared for communal Bat Mitzvahs,[37] but only three proceeded to the event; one was too nervous to go through the ritual.[38]

Jean and Stan were interested in art, visited galleries regularly, and supported young artists. They gradually collected works for their home, including paintings by Pro Hart and Charles Blackman. Stan had met a young Jewish refugee, Judy Cassab, who was to become one of Australia's best known female artists. Before she began her climb to success, she painted a portrait of Diana as a seven-year-old in 1953. Stan had hopes that Cassab would eventually paint portraits of the other three girls, but her commercial success both here and in London prevented this.[39] Judy Cassab went on to win two Archibald Prizes. She later painted Stan's portrait for the Royal Australasian College of Physicians.

Judy Cassab was a patient of Goulston's in the early years after her arrival in Sydney. In her published diaries, she describes her reactions to the enormous stresses that she and her husband were under then and the physical consequences that were severe enough to interrupt important travel. In an entry dated 3 July 1953, she described such an episode and wrote, 'I immediately ran to Dr Goulston who, last time, miraculously cured me in one visit'.[40] Her family stresses included financial ones, as this was some time before her portraits were selling well and before her husband had been able to carve out a new career. Judy and Stan remained friends and, in celebration of his ninetieth birthday, when Judy was eighty-five, he received from her a beautiful card which she had painted in watercolour.

Within and outside the family, observers were unanimous that the marriage of Jean and Stan was a remarkably happy one, with each partner supportive of the other.[41] That Stan was able to be so committed to his profession says much about the support and understanding that Jean and their daughters provided.[42] They were well aware that for Stan, 'his patients came first. Day and night they would ring and Dad was always available.'[43] That no marriage is perfect was recognised by Stan, who was able to admit in later life, 'naturally we quarrelled and we had times when we had different views on things'.[44]

With maturity, the girls gradually moved out of home and then away from Sydney. This distressed Jean considerably, while Stan was quite relaxed about it.[45] Jean may have recognised, and now regretted, that she had fostered in her daughters from a young age a positive attitude to travel and to seeing more of the world.[46]

Seeing the total commitment involved in their father's medical work, it is unsurprising that no daughter chose this professional path. They were encouraged to go to university and all obtained a tertiary education of their own choosing. Their parents did not seek to direct them; their main wish was for their daughters to have happy lives.[47] They were free to follow their real interests and, as a result, education in art, literature, science and social work resulted, with later diversions into other fields. While the girls' interests were all different, they were supportive of one another and no envy or disaffection ever surfaced.

Eventually each daughter left home to become independent, with two settling permanently in the USA, one in Melbourne and another in Mollymook. Stan and Jean kept in contact with them all by travelling when possible but also by frequent letter-writing, and, for Stan, by writing poetry and stories for his grandchildren. As all their grandchildren were distant, Sydney-based grand-nieces and nephews filled the gap. Without fail each year, Stan would travel to Melbourne to prune his daughter's roses.

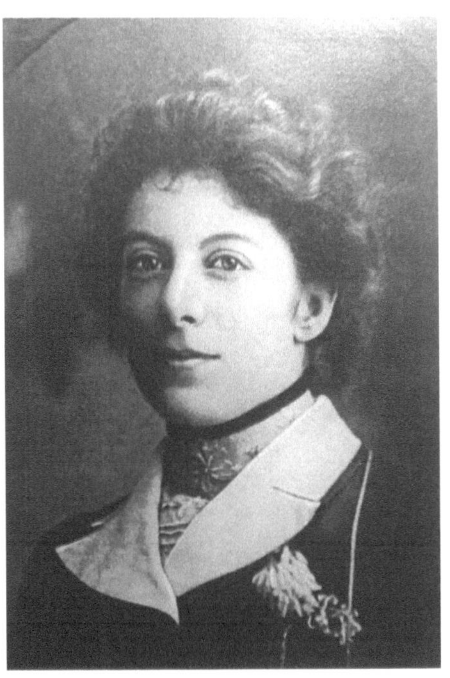

Left

Stan Goulston's mother,
Flora Wollff, circa 1902.

Below

John Goulston (on the left) with
Jacob Danglow, circa 1950.

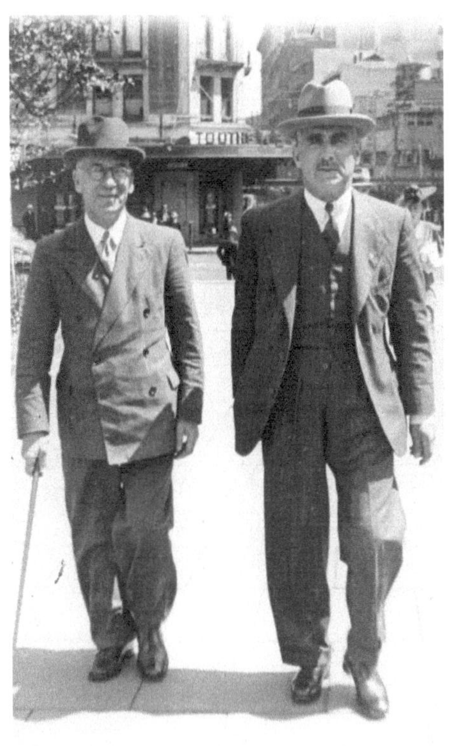

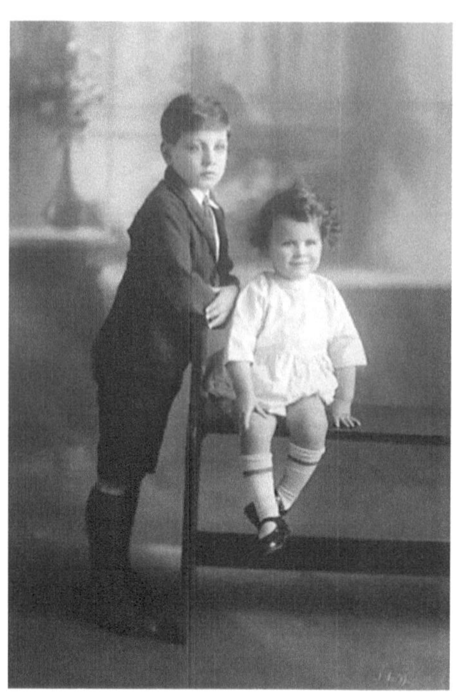

Left

Stan Goulston with sister Peggy, circa 1922.

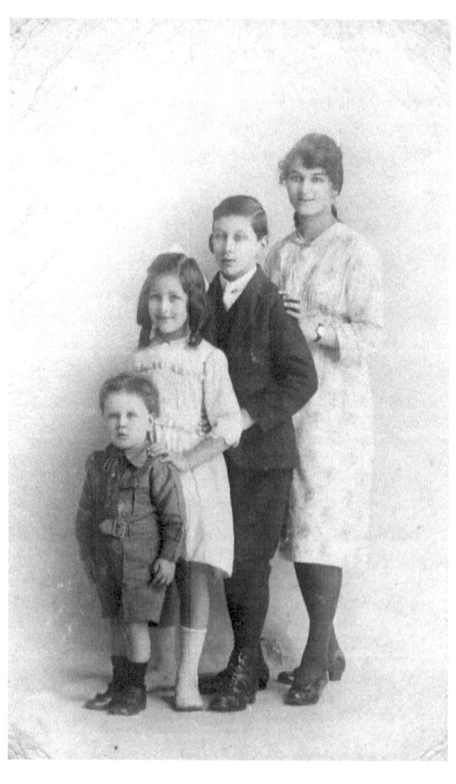

Below

Children of Flora and John Goulston: Stan, Edna, Eric and Olive, circa 1917.

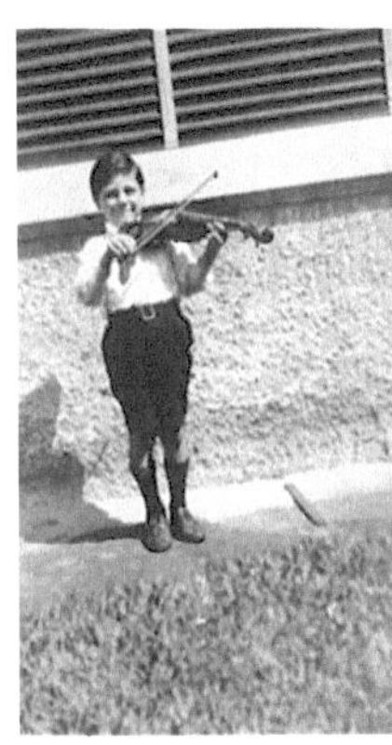

Left

Stan Goulston aged eight years, with violin.

Below

Resident medical officers at Royal Prince Alfred Hospital, 1939.

Bottom

Jean Danglow and Stan Goulston with their parents, on the occasion of the couple's engagement, 29 February 1940. Left to Right: Roy Goulston, Peggy Goulston, Jean Danglow, Stan Goulston, Golda Goulston, John Goulston, May Danglow and Jacob Danglow.

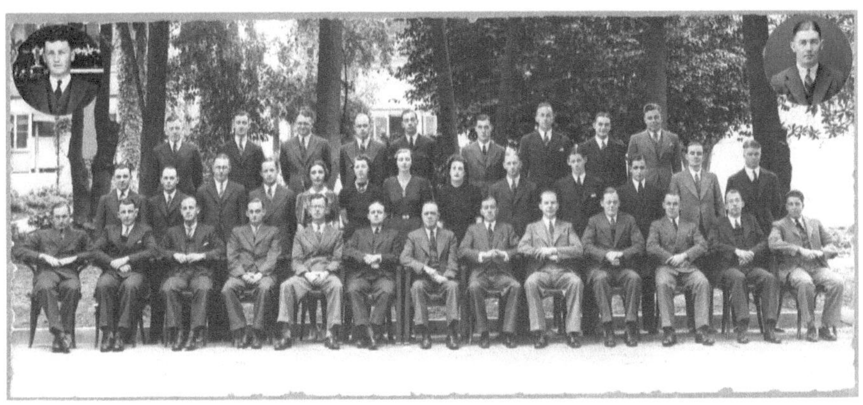

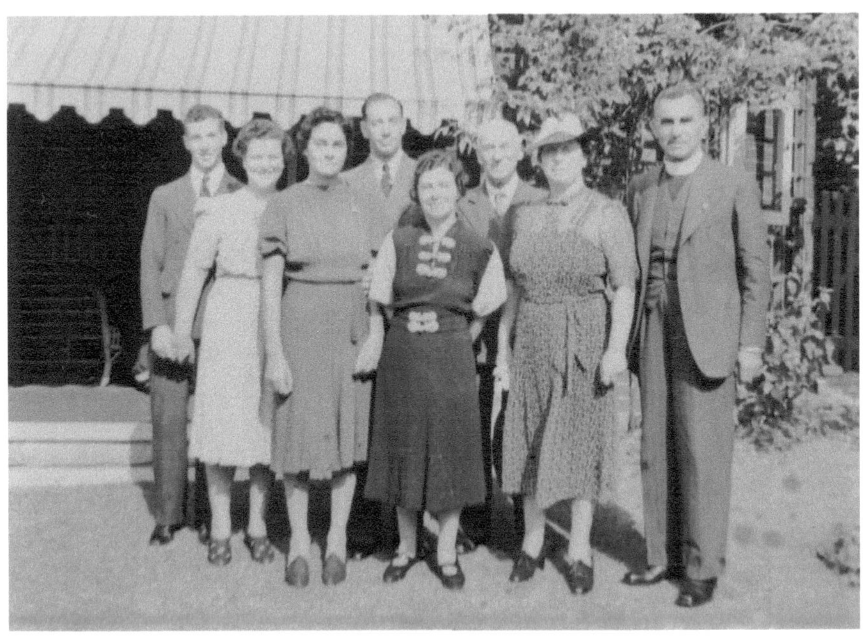

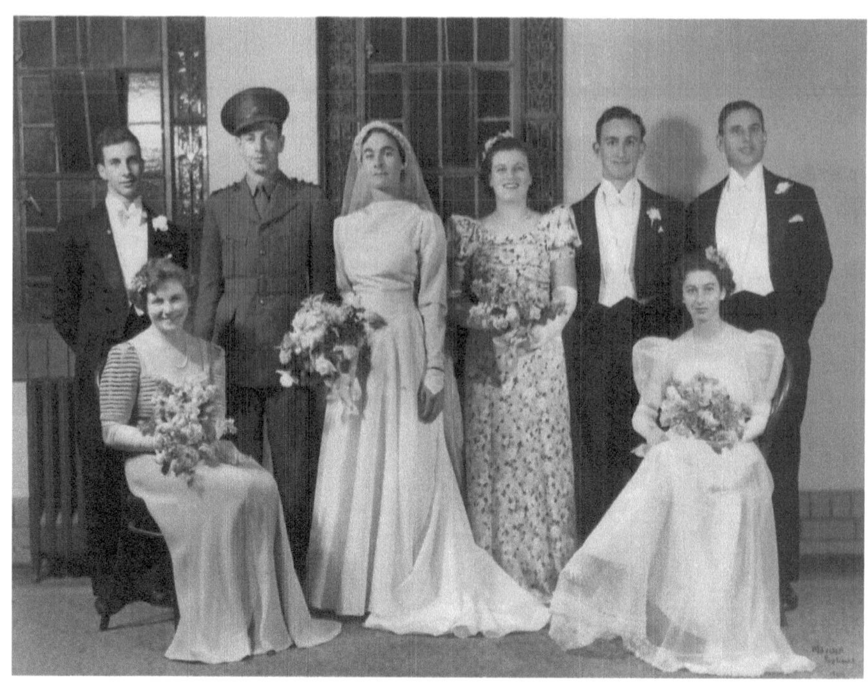

Jean and Stan Goulston and wedding party: Philippa Plottel, Peggy Goulston, Mary Michaelis, Roy Goulston, Frank Danglow and Leo Slutzkin, 25 May 1940.

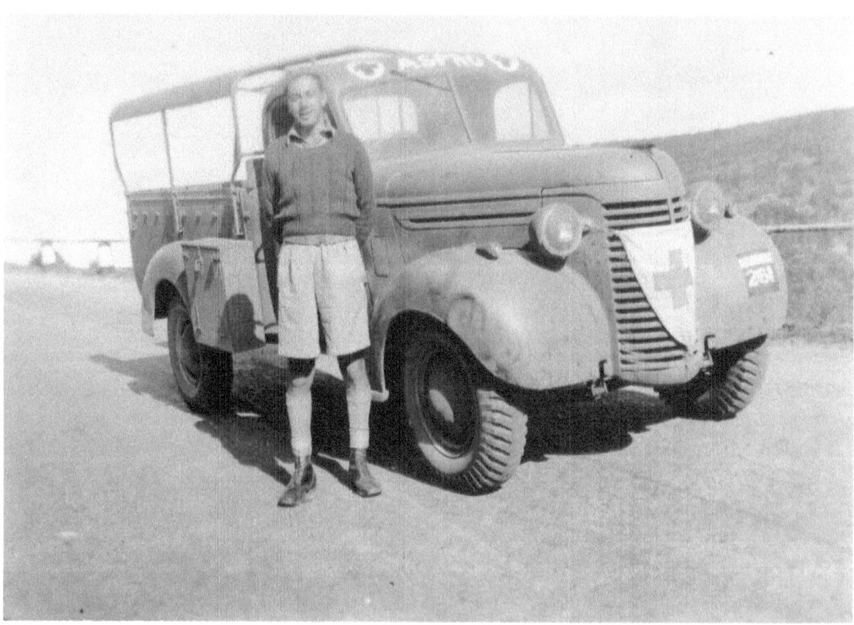

Captain Stan Goulston with his vehicle 'Aspro', Libya, 1941.

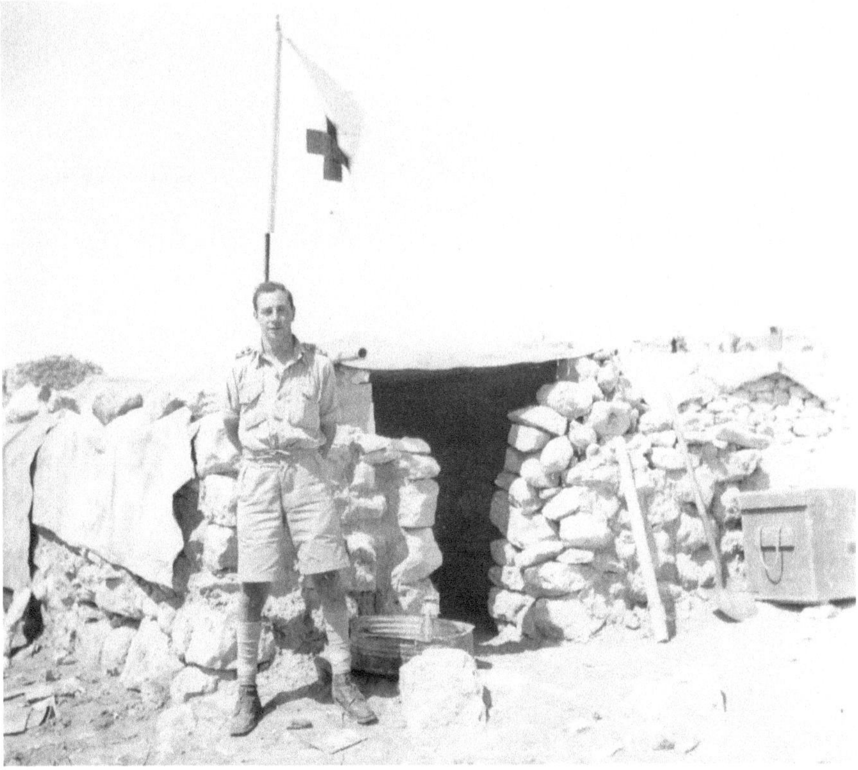

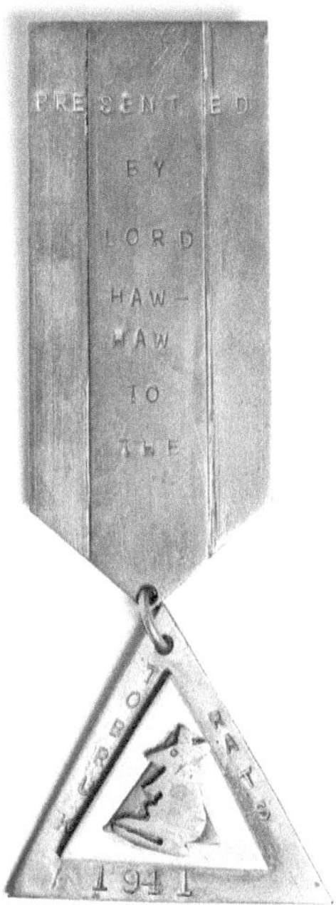

Above

Stan Goulston at a regimental aid post at Tobruk, 1941.

Left

Stan Goulston's 'Rats of Tobruk' medal.
(Courtesy Michael Wearne Photography)

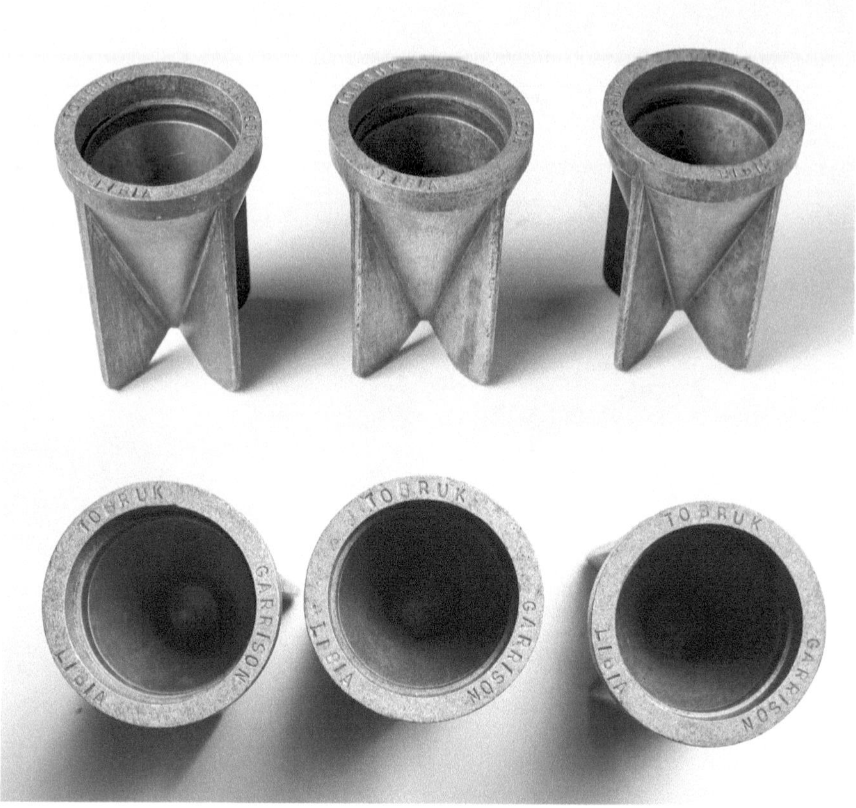

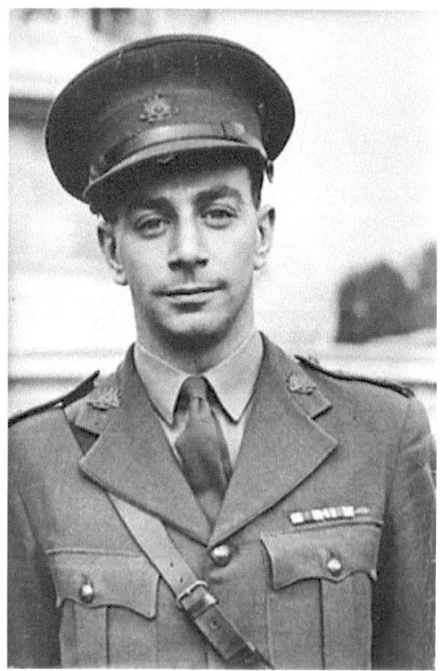

Above

Egg-cups made from Italian shells, presented to Captain Stan Goulston, Tobruk, 1941.

(Courtesy Michael Wearne Photography)

Left

Major Stan Goulston, AIF, on the day he received the Military Cross at Buckingham Palace, 10 October 1944.

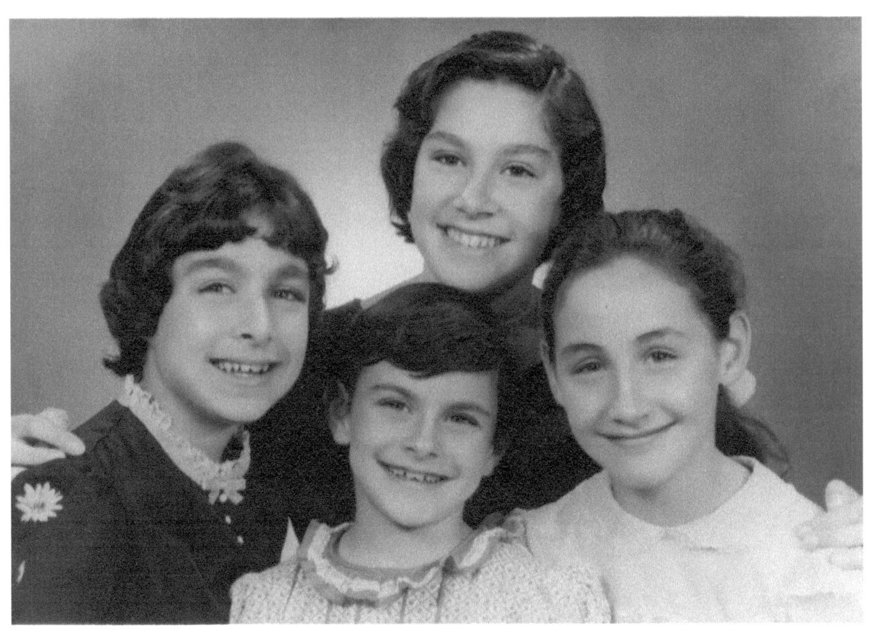

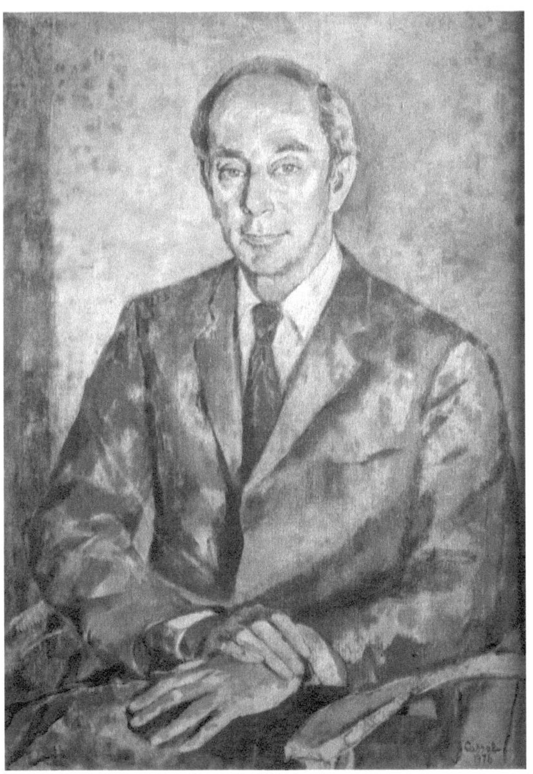

Above

Left to right: Diana, Sadhana, Wendy and Sue Goulston, circa 1960.

Left

Portrait of Stan Goulston painted by Judy Cassab, 1976.
(Reproduced with the permission of the RACP)

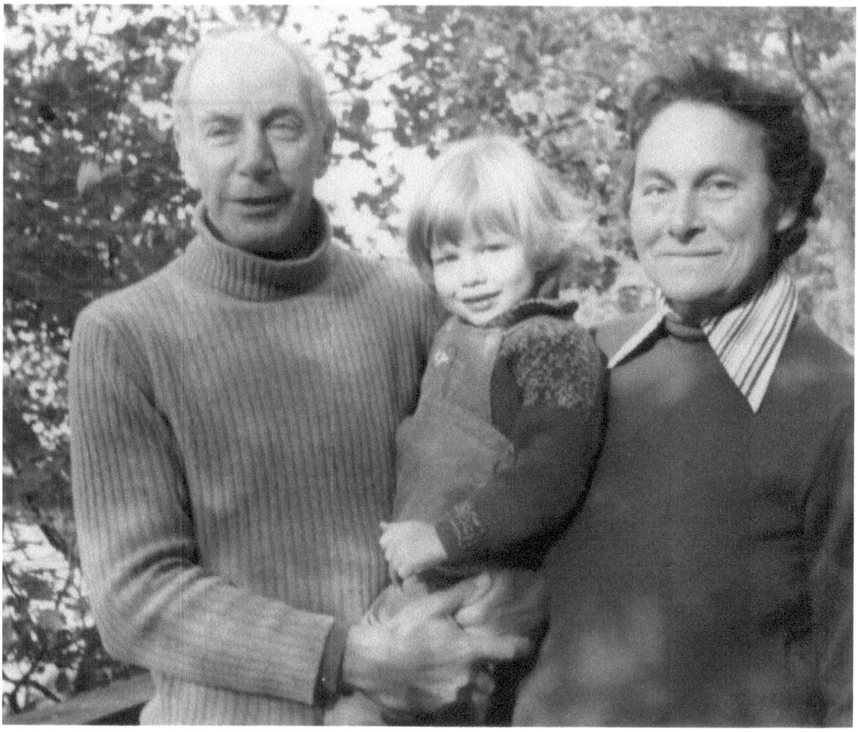

Stan and Jean Goulston with first grandson, James, 1978.

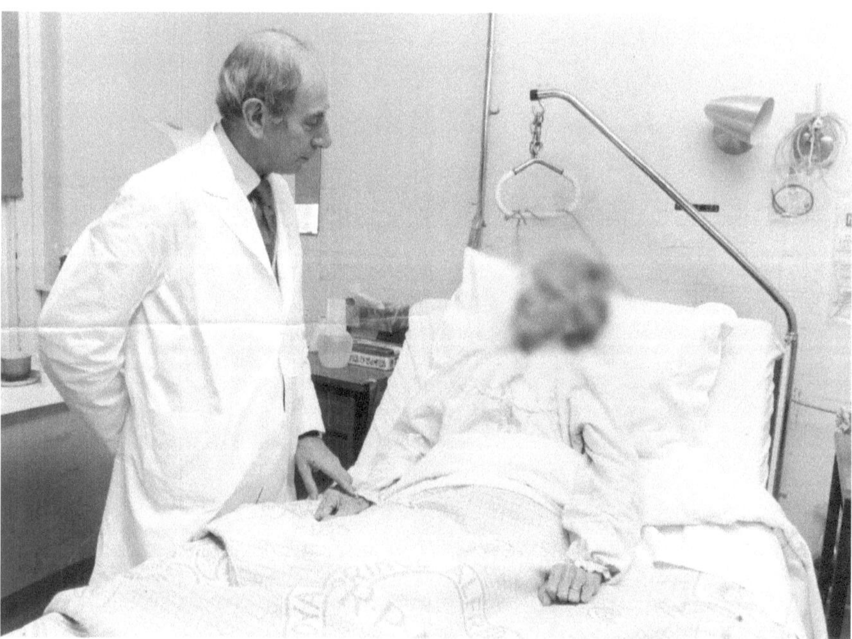

Stan Goulston at the bedside, Royal Prince Alfred Hospital, circa 1980.

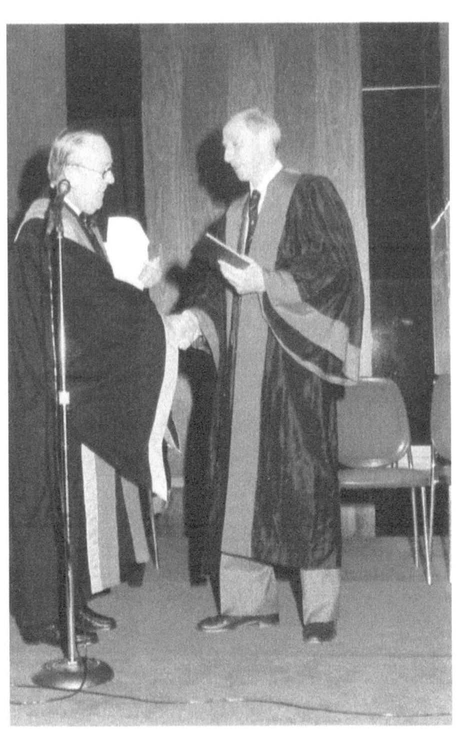

Left

Stan Goulston being presented with the Neil Hamilton Fairley Medal by RACP President, Dr Bryan Hudson, 1984.

Below

Stan Goulston receiving his Master of Philosophy degree from University of Sydney Chancellor, Dame Leonie Kramer, 1997.

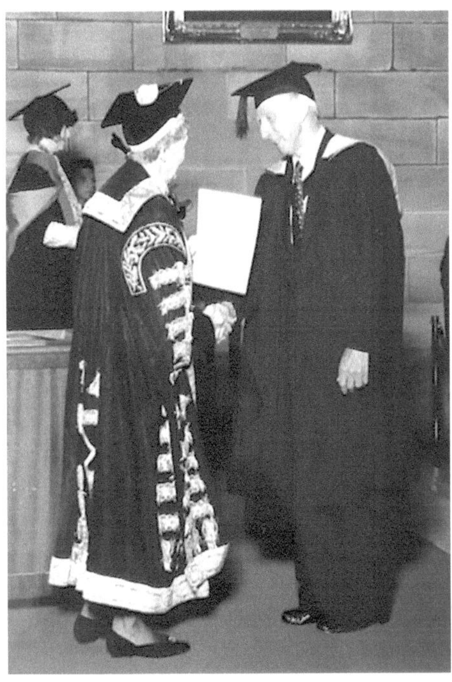

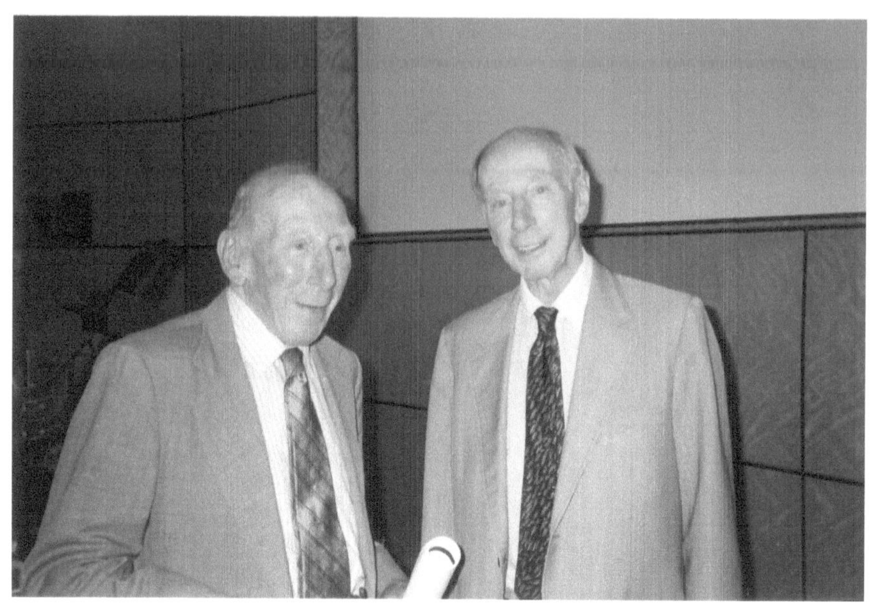

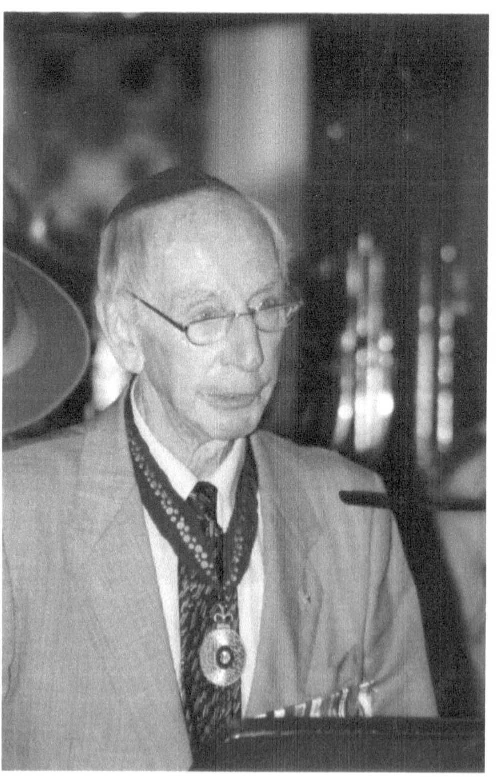

Above

Friends for life: Stan with brother Eric Goulston, 1995.

Left

Stan Goulston addressing the New South Wales Association of Jewish Service and Ex-Servicemen and Women, April 2002.

CHAPTER 7

Honorary Physician to the Royal Prince Alfred Hospital

Goulston joined the senior medical staff at the Royal Prince Alfred Hospital (RPAH) at a propitious time. As a result, he participated in an era of remarkable change and witnessed advances in virtually every field of medicine during his career. In 1947, the year of his appointment, the RPAH was already the largest teaching hospital in Australia. For justifiable reasons, its medical staff members were confident also that it was the finest hospital in the nation. Its proud record may be attributed in part to its physical situation adjacent to the University of Sydney and its close affiliation with the university.

Surprisingly, a formal history of the hospital is yet to be written but clear accounts of its establishment have been published.[1] In 1868, Prince Alfred, Duke of Edinburgh and second son of Queen Victoria, was in Sydney as the first member of the Royal Family to visit Australia. A deranged citizen of Irish origin sought to assassinate him. The Prince was wounded but recovered fully. The mortified citizens of Sydney decided to honour the Prince by building a new general hospital to be named after him. A public appeal readily raised the funds and the University of Sydney made suitable land available on its western border, with the stipulation that the hospital be a teaching hospital of the university. The new hospital, opened in 1882, was initially named the Prince Alfred Hospital with the prefix 'Royal' being added in 1903.

The University of Sydney did not establish a Faculty of Medicine until 1883. From then, the Hospital Board and the university jointly appointed the senior medical staff to the RPAH. The university was the first in Australia to create chairs in Medicine and in Surgery and full-time professors in both fields were appointed in the 1930 – G.C. Lambie in Medicine and Harold Dew in Surgery. The University of Sydney's rival, the University of Melbourne, had established a Faculty of Medicine in 1858 but lagged behind badly in promoting academic medicine; its first full-time professors in Medicine and Surgery were not appointed until well after World War II. At RPAH, some specialisation in surgery was recognised early in the twentieth century – including ear, nose and throat; eye; and gynaecology. To these specialisms were added orthopaedics and neurosurgery, the last in 1938.

Immediately after World War II, most patient care at RPAH was provided by general medical and general surgical units. Each general medical unit was headed by an honorary physician supported by an assistant honorary physician; the former looked after inpatients and the latter attended the outpatient clinics. This was a hierarchical system; an assistant honorary physician needed to wait until an honorary physician retired at the age of sixty before he (they were all men) could apply to be promoted. The unit structure was arranged so that each medical unit was paired with a surgical unit and referral to any other surgeon was not permitted. This system was designed to spread the workload evenly but, as general surgeons were gradually developing special skills in different fields, it was also a system that could deny a patient access to the best care. It was ready for change, and the hospital was about to appoint a physician whose clinical research into the illness of ulcerative colitis would drive this change.[2]

Before Goulston left London, he had made an application to the RPAH for an appointment as an honorary assistant physician. He would not have been aware who the other applicants were and was probably unaware that returned servicemen were likely to be favoured in any appointment process. He was aware that RPAH, and other Sydney hospitals, had suspended making new appointments of honorary physicians for the duration of the war. This was a wise approach,[3] as it ensured that physicians who volunteered to join the Armed Forces would not be disadvantaged.[4] He would have been cognisant that between his first fifteen months after graduation and his recent short period of training at Hammersmith, he had had six years away from general clinical medicine. He would also have been worried that in those six years, he might have been forgotten by his alma mater.

With all these considerations, he must have been concerned at his chances of appointment for a position that he had set his heart on. Towards the end of 1946, he asked a number of doctors to write letters of recommendation to the RPAH. Copies of the letters written on his behalf are still held by his family. They provide insight into the high regard in which he was already held and additionally offer detail about the people he had worked with and the responsibilities he had handled. It is worthwhile to pause and look at what these people wrote and, at the same time, appreciate how easy the task of the Appointments Board at RPAH must have been.

First, the letters from those doctors with whom Goulston had worked in London. In a letter dated 9 October 1946, Colonel John H. Anderson wrote:

> In 1944 Major Goulston MC, AAMC was specially selected and sent to London to act as Deputy Director General Medical Service on the Australian Army Staff and served as that from June 1944 to June 1946 … In that two years, Dr Goulston passed his Membership of the Royal College of Physicians of London at his first attempt; this was specially meritorious as any preparatory work had to be done in his scanty off duty hours … His appointment as Registrar at the British Postgraduate Medical School from June to Dec 1946 testifies to his worth as a physician … His work in London has brought him in frequent contact with many of the leaders

of British Medicine and he was liked and trusted by them both for his personal qualities and his professional judgment.[5]

Dr John McMichael on 2 November 1946 wrote that he had met Goulston in the latter days of the war as Medical Liaison Officer and noted:

> [H]e took a deep interest in the work we were doing at this school and was a frequent visitor on staff rounds … I quickly came to form a high opinion of his capacity and was delighted when he expressed his intention of spending some time at the school on the cessation of hostilities. As his interests lay rather in the field of gastroenterology, he has been attached to the service of Dr Sherlock and Dr Avery Jones where he has been doing excellent work.[6]

Professor (formerly Brigadier) Neil Hamilton Fairley, an Australian and recently appointed Head of the Department of Tropical Medicine at the University of London, wrote on 19 August 1946:

> I was in London on military duty in 1944 when Major Goulston took over for several months from the ADGMS, Col. J Anderson, and during this period I was most impressed with his personality and his quite outstanding achievements as an administrator and medical liaison officer … In June this year he was appointed Registrar at the British Postgraduate Medical School, Hammersmith, a much sought after appointment among the younger physicians in London.[7]

In the same month, Dr Sheila Sherlock wrote:

> [H]e first came here in June 45. On release from the Army in July 46, I was pleased to secure his service as my Senior Medical Registrar … He has a high sense of responsibility to

his patients and an excellent clinical acumen. He has himself started a study of the means of prolonging penicillin action. He has decided on a career in academic and consultative medicine.[8]

From the doctors with whom he had worked in Australia came similar glowing recommendations. Dr John Halliday[9] at RPAH regarded Goulston as 'one of the best house physicians I have ever had'. Dr W.P. MacCallum,[10] also a physician at RPAH, held the view that Goulston's 'record of achievement has been outstanding in every regard' and added:

> [H]e is a most efficient, conscientious and hard-working individual who combines a flair for administration with sound judgment, a capacity for taking infinite pains and a practical enthusiasm ... he has rendered service of the greatest value and has won golden opinions from all who have been associated with him.

Dr A.W. Morrow,[11] at the end of a strong letter, observed that 'during this period [in London] he [i.e., Goulston] was constantly in contact with many outstanding scientific personalities, an experience which is granted to few men of his age'. Dr Kempson Maddox[12] wrote that '[i]n spite of his divorcement from academic medicine he obtained both the MRACP and the MRCP while in Military Service – an unprecedented achievement'. And Dr Lorimer Dodds[13] and Dr Charles Kellaway[14] made equally positive comments.

He need not have worried, as the Hospital Board not only appointed Goulston as an Assistant Honorary Physician but he was listed as the 'first appointee'.[15] He was also the youngest of the four. Being the first appointed meant that if and when a more senior position became vacant, he would have the inside running for that position. The board made an excellent choice, as Goulston was to serve the hospital in an honorary capacity until his compulsory retirement at the age of sixty-five. For most of those years, he spent forty to fifty per cent of his working week at the hospital.[16] In his last few years on the staff at RPAH, there was agitation from some quarters for sessional payment but this was not introduced until 1980 – too late to benefit Goulston. This was never of concern to him, as he saw himself as privileged to be an honorary physician at such a fine hospital.[17]

Nevertheless it was a big sacrifice that honorary medical and surgical staff were making in terms of their income. In the 1940s, 1950s and 1960s, general practitioners were the doctors driving expensive cars. These were the years before Medibank and Medicare, and many patients could not afford to be referred to consultant physicians in private practice. At this time also, 'professional courtesy' was practised – meaning that consultant physicians, surgeons and obstetricians did not bill doctors or their family members.[18] Consultants at the 'top of the tree' set high fees for patients who could afford them and these doctors were prepared to spend part of their weekends travelling to country towns, at the request of general practitioners, with lucrative returns for seeing just two or three patients.[19]

What drove Goulston and many like him across Australia to accept such working conditions? Was it the satisfaction of sitting at the top of the profession? Was it giving back by teaching those who followed? Was it working in a stimulating and supportive environment with colleagues who were like-minded and available to provide advice when needed? To many it was an appreciation that a prestigious appointment was more likely to attract referrals from general practitioners. Being personally known as the teachers of medical students was an additional factor; in a year or two, these students would be in general practice and likely to refer patients to their teachers. There is no doubt that then, as now, it was at the teaching hospitals where advances in medicine (in the most general meaning of 'medicine') were made or first introduced, and it was and still is exciting to be part of such an environment. From reflections later in life, it seems that it was this last aspect in particular that led Goulston to want to be on the staff of RPAH.

Not that the hospital environment was perfect. When Goulston was first appointed, the Medical Board of the hospital (a strange name, as this was the equivalent of the Senior Medical Staff Association of other major hospitals) was dominated and controlled by the honorary visiting staff. The board would not permit any salaried, full-time appointees (and there were some in pathology and radiology) to belong to the association. In 1961, full-time salaried doctors were invited to attend meetings but it was to be another five years before they were given full voting rights. Assistant honorary physicians were 'kept in their place' by the more senior honorary physicians. An assistant only took responsibility for inpatients when his senior was on leave. It was said that the assistants were aware of the age and date of birth of their seniors – the suggestion being that they were impatiently waiting for their compulsory retirement.[20]

At the time of Goulston's first senior appointment, RPAH was well led by the chairman of the hospital board of directors, Dr (later Sir) Herbert Schlink.[21] Goulston saw him as a 'tough man, [a] very powerful man' for whom RPAH 'was his everything, he worked terribly hard'. Goulston recalled Schlink saying that every other hospital was 'terribly envious of RPAH and long may it continue, it is a great thing'.

Goulston's physician seniors when he was appointed in 1947 included three men who influenced him as role models and mentors. They were Dr (later Sir) Thomas Greenaway,[22] Dr William 'Billy' Bye[23] and Dr (later Sir) William Morrow. It is noteworthy that these three physicians were known for their commitment to their patients and to the hospital, their warmth in human relations, and their enthusiasm for teaching. Greenaway was also known for his punctuality, his appreciation of the need for specialisation and for his roles with the Royal Australasian College of Physicians (RACP). Bye was acknowledged especially for his humility and 'scorn for pretence'. Morrow was only twelve years older than Goulston and they were to become a powerful team in developing gastroenterology; their relationship is explored in a later chapter.

In time, Goulston as a physician became as admired and revered at RPAH as had been Greenaway and Bye. Trainee physicians who served under Goulston were unstinting in their praise. The characteristic that stood out was his gentle nature, with one trainee describing him as 'the most gentle person he ever met'.[24] A second characteristic was his humility, being described as 'one of the humblest and gentlest people'.[25] A third was his even-tempered disposition; he never seemed upset or irritated even with the most difficult of patients.[26] As a supervisor of young doctors, he was capable of quietly and gently showing displeasure if the need arose. He had a disarming approach of addressing a junior doctor as 'Boy', possibly when he was unsure of their name. This was never used in a demeaning or derogatory way.

As Clinical Superintendent at RPAH in 1969, Dr John Chalmers got to know Goulston well. Fifty years later he readily recalled what he admired in Goulston then. He saw him as 'a brilliant individual … a towering strength at PA – strong, silent yet warm' and 'never pushy'. He observed that Goulston never tried to promote his own cause and that his opinion was 'sought by all sorts of people'. As others had noted, Chalmers also saw Goulston as a modest and self-effacing person, one who was looked up to by all and who gave wise advice and 'unassuming guidance'.[27]

Colleagues over the years that followed were equally impressed. Miles Little, who first met Goulston while he, Miles, was still a medical student, and who subsequently became a professional colleague and friend, felt that Goulston 'radiated integrity', always went a little further than did his contemporaries to establish rapport with patients and students and was a 'truly exceptional teacher'.[28] Other former students warmly recalled his teaching.[29] Goulston also supported in other ways those medical students whom he was asked to instruct. One of his earliest students, Joachim Schneeweiss, warmly recalled their student group being invited for afternoon tea at the Goulston family home. A few months later, when Joachim suddenly fell ill at home with severe abdominal pain, he phoned Goulston for advice. Many years afterwards, in a letter of condolence to the Goulston family, Dr Schneeweiss, now a consultant physician, wrote that on that past occasion Dr Goulston came immediately to see him in his home in Bondi, diagnosed a perforated ulcer, gave a pain-killing injection and arranged for an ambulance to take him to hospital.[30]

Goulston developed a reputation for giving support to other doctors, especially those junior to him.[31] His advice was sought by so many that progress through the corridors of the hospital was frequently interrupted. Even when he was meant to be back in his private rooms, he was always patient and willing to listen.[32] If he walked with the person seeking advice, he fell in step with that person.[33]

Young doctors learned from observing his bedside manner, which was always respectful and empathic. They noted his thoroughness, his willingness to admit to not knowing things, his respect for nursing staff and his additional efforts in personally seeking out the pathologists, radiologists and surgeons to discuss his patients. Not only did young doctors desire to work on his ward but so too did other health professionals, such as social workers.

In 1960 he was promoted to Honorary Physician. His general medical ward was shared with another inpatient physician, Dr Richard Harris. Goulston at any one time would have sixteen to twenty patients in the ward, a mixture of people with gastroenterological and other medical problems. His working week as an honorary general physician involved two afternoon ward rounds – rounds that included patient care and informal teaching of his resident and registrar and a visit to pathology and radiology. In those days, ward rounds were a formal occasion, as he was always greeted at the ward by the senior nurse and the round began with a cup of tea and a sandwich. The senior nurse then accompanied the round.

Goulston taught a group of medical students each week, usually separately from the ward round. On Friday afternoons he was at the hospital from 1 p.m. onwards for educational meetings, finishing with Grand Rounds late in the afternoon. In his general medical role, he was always available to take telephone calls for advice from his registrar. However, he usually had relatively experienced registrars, on rotations of six months, and was comfortable to delegate to them patient care including initiating urgent specialist referrals.

Goulston willingly contributed to the teaching of trainee physicians preparing for the RACP examinations, conducting weekly teaching rounds for this purpose attended not only by RPAH registrars but by many from other Sydney hospitals.[34] His gentle style put the trainees at ease; as one participant described, he 'tested our understanding and revealed our ignorance without stress'.[35] His teaching rounds were compared favourably with those conducted at the Sydney Hospital by physician and college censor, Dr Alan McGuinness, whose fearsome reputation was known by trainees well beyond Sydney.

In the late 1950s, in addition to his general medical unit duties and his role in gastroenterology, Goulston served as an honorary part-time Senior Lecturer in the University of Sydney academic Department of Medicine based at RPAH, now led by Professor Ruthven Blackburn. Here he also had a clinical role. One junior doctor, whose first rotation after graduation in 1959 was in Blackburn's service, saw Goulston as the steadying influence on an otherwise temperamental group of physicians. That junior doctor, when a medical student in Blackburn's unit, had already been the beneficiary of Goulston's kindness.[36]

In Goulston's era there was little or no discussion of the qualities desired of a 'good doctor', so he would not have been familiar with the modern rehearsal of a long list of such qualities, even though he epitomised all of them. They now include such aspects as good communication skills, empathy, compassion, veracity and collegiality.[37] When asked in an interview in 2008 what he thought makes a good doctor, Goulston's immediate answer was 'to keep an open mind because patients come from all walks of life, even criminals. As a doctor, you can't judge them.' The question had arisen shortly after a discussion of his Army experience and his response suggests that his view of the world had been broadened by the experience. He was deeply aware of the importance of communication, empathy and compassion in medical practice, as we shall see in Chapter 12.

From a young age, Goulston was a keen observer of human nature and behaviour and this continued in the hospital setting. He set junior doctors a fine example of humility, modesty and quietly spoken gentle consistency. He never openly expressed criticism of his peers. Based on a poem written much earlier but not published until 2007, those peers were fortunate that he kept his views to himself. It was entitled 'Hospital Grand Rounds' and read as follows:

The weekly traditional pilgrimage,
The lecture theatre benches,
The sanctum sanctorum;
Staff, students congregate
Academics centre stage.

Live patients not admitted
Where once were welcomed
With courtesy, politeness and respect.
Now learned doctors gather
To solve problems so submitted

Identified by slides on screen,
Personal details, test results,
ECGs, MRIs
Somehow detached from reality
And what empathy might mean
Experts press narrow notions
Quote research from latest journals
Displaying one-up-man-ship.
A certain sibling rivalry
Expressing disparate emotions

Sitting in the audience I ponder
How to restore the patient's narrative
The meaning of the illness
Understanding of suffering
The balance of science and wondering?

To reshape Grand Rounds
Endless possibilities;
A doctor's string quartet?
The art of Arthur Boyd

Towards the healing of open wounds?

An appropriate literary resource
To illuminate and illustrate
Fundamental human problems?
Prose and poetry renderings
To supply and create a tour de force?

I creep away, leave the scene,
Drive to the sea, feel the wind,
Absorb the sun and listen to
The calming chatter of the birds.
Peace prevails where pandemonium prevailed.

As did most honorary physicians, Goulston happily taught a generation of medical students and regularly served as a clinical examiner for the Sydney University, again all without being paid. He also had honorary commitments in gastroenterology at the hospital and had to conduct a private practice to be able to support his family. For his private practice, initially he rented consulting rooms at 135 Macquarie Street – rooms that he later described as being dingy and in a ricketty old building that hosted a well-known abortionist one floor above and a 'fertility expert' in the office adjacent to Goulston's. His first patient, a male, 'walked off the street', unreferred, bringing a surprise diagnosis. The man complained of a sore throat and when Goulston examined his throat he saw the typical ulcers of secondary syphilis. The man refused to attend the Health Department so Goulston reluctantly began a series of penicillin injections. Halfway through treatment, the patient disappeared. His account was never paid. Goulston 'put it down to experience'.[38]

He soon recognised that travel to and from RPAH in Camperdown was an inefficient use of his time and he relocated to consulting rooms that had been built by the RPAH at 100 Carillon Avenue, Newtown. Now he had less than 200 metres to walk from his rooms to the hospital. Like his seniors, he too undertook some private consulting in rural New South Wales at weekends, flying to those centres.

In 1980, because of the rules of the day, he retired from his honorary appointments at RPAH.[39] He was still seen at the hospital, as he was made an Honorary Consultant Physician (a title akin to the university term, 'Emeritus'). He was always welcome to attend Grand Rounds and the weekly educational events in the Gastroenterology Department and he did so regularly. He continued to perform gastroscopies in the department[40] and remained in active private practice for many years. The educational events at RPAH were of importance to the clinical elements of his professional life, as well as to his role of chairing the Australian Drug Evaluation Committee (see Chapter 11) which was to continue for a number of years.

Recalling that he had played a large part in the commencement of specialisation in medicine at RPAH, he may have disagreed with a decision taken by the RPAH physicians at a retreat held at Bowral in the late 1980s. Here it was decided that the general medical units would be disbanded and all inpatients beds would be allocated to specialties, including that of geriatrics.[41] As a strong supporter of general medicine, he would have found this upsetting. Many other hospitals around Australia followed this precedent, but not all.[42]

CHAPTER 8

Gastroenterology and the Gastroenterological Society of Australia

Stan Goulston trained as a physician at a time when all physicians appointed to the senior medical staff of major teaching hospitals in Australia were honorary general physicians and were expected to cover the entire range of internal medicine. To emphasise how wide this range was, it included the following fields now handled by specialists: cardiology, dermatology, diabetes, endocrinology, gastroenterology, haematology, immunology, infectious diseases, nephrology, neurology, oncology, respiratory medicine and rheumatology. In the 1940s, some of these fields did not exist; nevertheless patients attended those hospitals with the illnesses now included under one or more of these categories.

Prior to World War II and following it, there was a gradual move to specialisation, first seen in surgery (e.g., orthopaedics and neurosurgery) and then in medicine. In the UK, this occurred through general physicians taking a particular interest in a field such as cardiology or neurology and becoming known for their expertise. However, all of these physicians still practised as generalists. Australian medicine closely followed British medicine, lagging behind a little. This model persisted in Australia in both hospitals and private practice until the 1970s. In private practice, it was driven by economics; consultant physicians depended on referrals from general practitioners and to refuse to see patients other than in the field of your special interest would lead to significant financial disadvantage – especially in the era before Medicare. In the teaching hospitals, there was an additional factor preventing the evolution of specialists: access to beds. The general physicians (and general surgeons) were the only senior medical staff who had a bed allocation and this was jealously guarded. As will be seen, the efforts to develop the specialty of gastroenterology ran into this obstruction at Royal Prince Alfred Hospital (RPAH).

For most of his practising life at RPAH, Goulston remained a general physician.[1] His general physician peers at RPAH who had special expertise in other areas did the same.[2] A prime example was Dr John Sands,[3] who graduated two years after Goulston and ran a general medical unit at RPAH in the 1960s. His special interest was in renal medicine and he contributed to the development of his specialty at RPAH in a manner similar to Goulston in gastroenterology. However, Goulston was unusual for his time in that he was more than a general physician with an interest in gastroenterology. He was also one of a small group of pioneer gastroenterologists who helped to pave the way for the over seven hundred gastroenterologists who now practise in Australia.[4] He did this by several means. He led by example as a clinical researcher in the field; he helped to establish the first gastroenterology unit in the nation;[5] he played a central role in the formation of the Gastroenterological Society of Australia (GESA). Here I examine his part in the establishment of Australia's first gastroenterology unit and then his role in the formation of GESA. His clinical research contributions are the subject of Chapter 9.

Goulston was stimulated by what he observed at Hammersmith Hospital in London in 1945 and 1946, where Dr Francis Avery-Jones was effectively a full-time gastroenterologist and where Dr Sheila Sherlock was embarking on her journey to becoming the best known hepatologist of her era. Perhaps by chance because a vacancy arose or perhaps because he sensed that Avery-Jones was past the peak of his eminent career, Goulston wisely obtained his introduction to his chosen specialty by working with Sherlock. However, he had no intention of restricting his field to diseases of the liver – as was evidenced by his purchase of a Herman Taylor gastroscope in London to bring back to Sydney. Once back in Australia, his initial clinical research efforts reflected his time with Sherlock,[6] but later his research interests broadened considerably.

Aware that the career of a consultant physician then was almost entirely dependent upon first holding an honorary appointment in general medicine at a teaching hospital, he sought and gained an appointment at RPAH, as described in the previous chapter. From this base, he had a chance of developing further as a gastroenterologist and building the type of unit that he had seen in action at Hammersmith. Fortunately he had a more senior physician at RPAH with the same vision, Dr Bill (later Sir William) Morrow. As will be seen, the career paths of Morrow and Goulston were similar, with Goulston following in some of Morrow's footsteps. Morrow was twelve years senior to Goulston, so it is likely that Morrow was a supporter, mentor and role model for Goulston.

Morrow was born in 1903 in East Maitland, New South Wales.[7] He attended Newington College[8] in Sydney, presumably as a boarder, where he thrived academically (he was dux of the school) and at sport. Like Goulston later, he won an exhibition at the Leaving Certificate examinations and went to Sydney University to study medicine. He graduated with first-class honours in 1927.[9]

He served as a Junior Resident Medical Officer at RPAH in 1927 and continued his training there as a Medical Registrar and then as Deputy Clinical Superintendent in 1932.[10] In 1933 he went to London, where he sat and passed the membership examination for the Royal College of Physicians (he was made a Fellow in 1949). He returned to Sydney and in 1934 was appointed an Honorary Assistant Physician at RPAH. He became a foundation member of the Royal Australasian College of Physicians (RACP) when it was established in 1938.

In 1929, Morrow had joined the Sydney University Regiment of the Citizens Military Force and was made a Captain. After war broke out, he enlisted in the Australian Imperial Force in 1940 and was promoted to Lieutenant Colonel in the Australian Army Medical Corps (AAMC). In May 1940 he joined the 2nd/5th Australian General Hospital (AGH). His team sailed for the Middle East in October 1940. In April 1941, the 2nd/5th AGH was part of the disastrous campaign[11] in Greece and they were forced to evacuate to Crete and eventually back to Egypt. In the course of the evacuation, his commanding officer was killed and Morrow had to take command of the 2nd/5th AGH. As recorded later by a former junior colleague,[12] Morrow was awarded the Distinguished Service Order (DSO) for 'his leadership, organisation and calmness in the face of enemy aerial attacks' during the evacuation.[13] Like Stan Goulston, Morrow was also 'mentioned in dispatches' during his war service.

He returned to Australia in March 1942 and held a number of senior posts with the AAMC until he was transferred to the Officers Reserve list at the end of 1945. Free to return to civilian life, he took up his previous appointment as Honorary Assistant Physician at RPAH. He was promoted to Honorary Physician in 1951. During these years, he also conducted a private practice and held visiting appointments at the Repatriation General Hospital at Concord and at district hospitals. In 1948 he was awarded a travel fellowship and visited gastroenterology centres in the USA and UK. He returned with the desire to see a gastroenterology service established at RPAH.

On return from his 1948 travels, Morrow was able to convince the RPAH to form a Gastroenterology Unit (GE Unit).[14] It had an inauspicious start, as the hospital allocated the new unit one basement room but no hospital beds. This was to be a consultative service[15] from day one. In addition to consulting when requested on inpatients, the new unit aimed to train future gastroenterologists and to conduct research.

Morrow was by now well connected as a member of the exclusive Australian Club,[16] where he served a term as the club president. He was said to have developed a close relationship with a fellow member, the Governor General of Australia, Sir William Slim, after Slim's arrival in Australia in 1953.[17] Morrow was knighted in 1959, for services to medicine and the community,[18] at the relatively young age of fifty-three and this may have assisted him with social connections. He also had as a close friend[19] and benefactor a successful businessman, Philip Bushell.[20] Bushell had established the Bushell Trust with a major aim of supporting medical education and research. The trust initially donated funds to allow the employment of a registrar and a secretary for the nascent GE Unit and continued to provide generous support for many years. And Morrow had a keen young colleague, Stan Goulston, to help build the new service.

Some of the many other duties that Morrow took on during his career included lecturing in therapeutics to medical students at Sydney University, chairing the Postgraduate Committee of Medicine of the university and serving as a member, and later the chair, of the Australian Drug Evaluation Committee of the Federal Health Department. Morrow was a foundation member of the RACP and served the college as Censor-in-Chief and as President. He was the Foundation President of GESA. And eventually the gastroenterology service that he founded at RPAH was named after him. He died in 1977, at the age of seventy-four.

Morrow was highly regarded as a caring and competent physician.[21] He was described by one of his trainees as a 'real gentleman' and an excellent calm, confident physician with a good bedside manner who treated everyone with respect.[22] He was an enthusiastic teacher who for many years conducted a teaching round to assist candidates for the Membership of the Royal Australasian College of Physicians (MRACP) examinations. He was not held to have an academic bent, in contrast to the views held about Goulston, but the two got on well as professional colleagues.[23] Morrow was seen as more outgoing, while some trainees found Goulston more reserved and thus they were less sure of where they stood with him.

Goulston described Morrow as one of three senior physicians at RPAH who influenced his approach to medicine, but there must have been more to this successful partnership. Morrow was about the same age as Goulston's elder brother Eric, so perhaps Morrow was a role model as well as a colleague. In addition, Morrow had access to vital funds without which the formation of a gastroenterology service may have been delayed many years. Observers noted that Goulston always deferred to Morrow and was comfortable to be a loyal deputy.[24] Trainees were impressed by Goulston as an excellent teacher at the bedside, as was Morrow. They were regarded as very good doctors who worked well as a team.[25] Away from work, apart from the monthly journal club hosted of an evening, initially at Bill Morrow's home, Goulston and Morrow moved in separate social circles.[26]

As an enthusiastic team, Morrow and Goulston set about building the new service. Funds from the Bushell Trust enabled the hiring first of a secretary, Jan Edwards, and then in 1950 a full-time Registrar, Dr Brian Billington. The service was provided with a single large basement room that sat under the original hospital building. It had previously been the hospital sewing or linen room and it had no windows. In the middle of the room sat a large table that filled much of the available space.[27] That table served as the work desk for the secretary, the registrar and a dietician who had a joint appointment with the GE Unit and the Clinical Research Unit (CRU). Later, when a second registrar was appointed, the table accommodated him readily as well.[28] Entrance to the large room was via a short passage off which sat a second, much smaller room, again without a window. This served as the examination room, although it had no facilities – not even a washbasin.

Initially the range of services offered by the GE Unit was restricted to clinical consultations and a Monday morning gastroscopy session conducted in the operating theatres. From the outset, the unit possessed two gastroscopes – the Herman Taylor instrument[29] that Goulston had brought from London and a Schindler instrument[30] donated by the ear, nose and throat surgeons. The team was cohesive and collaborative from the start, as Morrow and Goulston jointly attended the Monday gastroscopy session with their registrar, after which the group would visit the Radiology Department to review the week's X-rays and the Pathology Department to review the findings of liver and other biopsies. They would end the morning by joining Ruthven Blackburn for a cup of tea in the CRU.

From the outset there was a form of symbiosis between the GE Unit and the CRU. The latter had been established in 1949 with Dr Ruthven Blackburn as its full-time Director. Blackburn graduated three years ahead of Goulston and won first place in his graduating year. He trained as a junior doctor at RPAH and enlisted in the Army in 1940, serving at first in the Middle East and then in New Guinea (today's Papua New Guinea). He was made a Lieutenant Colonel and Commanding Officer of the Army's Medical Research Unit in Cairns, working alongside Neil Hamilton Fairley on the control of malaria. After the war, he spent a year as a Rockefeller Foundation Fellow at Columbia University in New York and on his return received the CRU appointment at RPAH. He went on to an illustrious career, culminating in the award of Companion of the Order of Australia (AC)[31] on Australia Day in 2006. The citation for the award read: 'For service to the development of academic medicine and medical education in Australia, particularly in relation to the evolving relationship between research and clinical practice, and as a mentor influencing the professional development of a generation of leading health care professionals'.[32]

The CRU was also given basement accommodation with space for around fourteen beds. Because of the slope of the land on which the main hospital block sat, the space did have windows. Blackburn's clinical and research interests included liver disease. He was on good terms with Goulston and they cooperated closely from the start. As the two services grew, a joint appointment of a second registrar was made. In addition, there was movement of trainees between the two services. For example, an early trainee was Dr Jim Rankin, who in 1957 was appointed by Blackburn as a second Registrar but his duties were divided equally between the CRU and the GE Unit. He served alongside the GE Unit Registrar, Dr Dick Boden. The next year, Rankin replaced Boden as full-time Registrar to the GE Unit while in 1960 he was back in the CRU as its full-time Registrar. By 1961 he was a Research Fellow in the CRU before heading to the USA to gain additional research experience.

In 1957 Blackburn was appointed the Bosch Professor of Medicine at the University of Sydney, an appointment that made him Head of the university's Department of Medicine at RPAH. He now had a department, a clinical service and a research endeavour to run as well as the CRU. The links to the GE Unit were maintained – a relationship reinforced by the mutual respect and friendship enjoyed by Goulston and Blackburn. However, eventually Blackburn stepped down from his CRU role and the day-to-day connections between the two units gradually declined.

During these early years, a number of young general physicians on the honorary staff at RPAH served for a year in the GE Unit. They included Dr John Sands and Dr Frank Harding Burns. As these men went on to become specialists in other fields, their work in the GE Unit seems anomalous by today's approach to physician training. It can be explained by the expectation of RPAH that every honorary physician be competent across the entire field of general medicine. While these young appointees had passed the MRACP examination, they were keen to obtain a broad clinical experience and were happy to rotate across several areas while awaiting promotion. By spending a year in the GE Unit, which now had an outpatient clinic, these physicians were able to become familiar more rapidly with managing clinical problems such as peptic ulcer, chronic liver disease, various types of colitis and coeliac disease.

In the early 1950s, Goulston sought out a pathologist recently appointed to the RPAH, New Zealand graduate, Dr Vincent McGovern, to suggest that McGovern might take a special interest in what Goulston called 'the living tissues' – the biopsies of the liver, small intestine and rectum that were now available from the patients seen by the GE Unit. McGovern readily accepted the suggestion and thus began thirty years of close collaboration between the two men. The impact of their collaboration, especially in clinical research, is covered in the next chapter.

Collaboration with surgical colleagues was vital to Morrow and Goulston as well. As also discussed in more depth in the next chapter, Goulston and colleagues had become aware of the poor outcome for patients with severe ulcerative colitis. They had come to the conclusion that better results would depend on sooner surgical intervention and surgery being in the hands of only one or two expert surgeons. They identified surgeon Norman Wyndham for this task and Wyndham invited David Glenn to be his understudy.[33] The identification of a single surgeon in this manner contradicted official hospital policy but, through the presentation of thorough clinical research data and by quiet persuasion, Morrow and Goulston got their way.

From the outset, the GE Unit was active in medical education. Staff presented at the weekly medical grand rounds and at the annual hospital postgraduate week. The unit initiated Saturday morning case presentations attended by physicians from other Sydney hospitals. These were so popular that other specialist units joined and the GE Unit staff then only presented every four weeks or so. When the GE Unit relocated to a much larger area in 1961 and there was space for a clinical meeting, regular Monday 5 p.m. case presentations were held, attended by all members of the unit and supported by their pathology and radiology colleagues.

After the retirement of Morrow in 1963,[34] Goulston became the Honorary Physician in charge of the GE Unit, now renamed the A.W. Morrow Department of Gastroenterology. Goulston continued the practice of taking his junior medical staff (and sometimes, medical students) with him to look at and discuss pathology findings with Dr McGovern and his assistants and to visit the Radiology Department to view X-ray films and discuss their interpretation with Dr David Stephen and Dr Janet McCredie. Trainee physicians were impressed by this approach, which was novel to them as it was often mentioned in interviews many years later, as were other aspects of role-modelling as discussed in Chapter 7.

The relationship between the GE Unit staff with the radiologists and colorectal surgeons deserves more emphasis as it reflects well on all parties. Before the advent of fibre-optic endoscopy, the Morrow Unit physicians were dependent on high-quality radiological assessment of the gastrointestinal (GI) tract and the radiologists at RPAH did not let them down. When Dr Janet McCredie joined the Radiology Department in 1965, she was asked to specialise in GI radiology. She deeply valued the accessibility of the physicians and their willingness to drop what they were doing to attend the department. She still vividly recalls the immediate help she received from Stan Goulston when she telephoned him about her recognising tell-tale radiological evidence of chronic amoebic colitis.[35]

Aspiring young colorectal surgeon, Brian Morgan, had even more reason to respect and value the support of Morrow and Goulston. Morgan attended a conference in Boston in 1969 where he saw the newly released original fibre-optic colonoscope, a diagnostic instrument manufactured by ACMI.[36] He was so enthused that he placed an order for the instrument, priced at US $10,000. When he returned to RPAH, the medical administrators assessed the device as a gimmick and refused to fund it. Morgan turned to Morrow and Goulston in the GE Unit, who not only welcomed the new instrument but allocated Morgan time and space in their unit to gain experience with the new device. They also funded its purchase.[37] Morgan's innovative work using mannitol bowel washouts was facilitated by Nancy Perrott, an experienced trained nurse, whose primary appointment in the GE Unit was to perform gastric cytology after gastric lavage.[38] Morgan also deeply appreciated the ongoing support in this new endeavour that he received from Goulston.[39]

The growth of the GE Unit in the 1950s was slow but steady. Other investigative methods, clinical and laboratory, were introduced. In 1961 the unit was relocated to a more spacious area vacated by cardiology. The Bushell Trust provided funds to enable the appointment in 1960 of Australia's first full-time salaried gastroenterologist, Dr Alan Skyring. Consistent with the hospital politics of the day,[40] Dr Skyring's appointment was as Research Director whereas in practice, he ran the day-to-day affairs of the unit. Although Skyring, like Morrow, was more extrovert than Goulston, he had a good working relationship with Goulston. Just before Skyring took up his appointment, Goulston was awarded a Pfizer Travelling Scholarship by the RACP and in 1960 was able to visit leading gastroenterology centres in the USA, UK and Europe.

The GE Unit could now take on not only the training each year of a new clinical registrar but could also be home to one or more research fellows. Some but not all of the research output of these early fellows is described in Chapter 9. Much of the clinical research that Goulston was undertaking with his colleagues was original, and some of it led to changes in practice with striking improvement in patient outcomes. Their careful analysis of the outcomes of patients undergoing surgery for severe ulcerative colitis is a good example (see Chapter 9).

By the late 1960s, the A.W. Morrow Department of Gastroenterology was flourishing. Stan Goulston's status as the Australian gastroenterologist with the greatest expertise in ulcerative colitis was acknowledged when, at the 1969 annual meeting of GESA in Brisbane, he shared the seminar podium with two international visitors, surgeon Brian Brooke[41] from the UK and physician Burrill Crohn[42] from the USA.

Other teaching hospitals around Australia were envious of the Morrow Unit's reputation. Gradually similar units were established across the nation but none could claim that they were the first. The only competitor was the Clinical Research Unit headed by Dr (later Sir) Ian Wood at the Royal Melbourne Hospital, a joint activity with the Walter and Eliza Hall Institute. In reality, Wood's unit was never a specialised gastroenterology unit. However, there was such mutual respect and collaboration between the two services, including an exchange of registrars for one week each year, that Morrow and Goulston never sought to make a claim of precedence. Indeed the two men sought unsuccessfully to have Sir Ian Wood agree to be the Foundation President of GESA, the history of which is briefly discussed below.

In 1983, when the Department of Gastroenterology was rehoused on the eleventh floor of the new hospital block at RPAH, the staff honoured Goulston by commissioning his photographic portrait. It hangs in the entrance hall alongside an earlier portrait of Sir William Morrow. It was unveiled in the same week that Goulston received an Honorary Doctorate of Medicine from the University of Sydney.[43]

Goulston remained a member of the Morrow Department until 1991. For all these years, he was a regular attendee at the educational events at RPAH, including the Monday afternoon clinical meetings of the department. When he stepped back, colleagues from the Morrow Unit, past and present, gave a dinner in his honour, held at St John's College, University of Sydney. Among the seventy or so attendees were the original unit secretary, Jan Scott-Miller (née Edwards), and several of the early registrars, as well as nurses, surgeons, pathologists and radiologists with whom Stan had worked so closely. Family members, his brother Eric and nephew Dr Kerry Goulston, were also present. His wife Jean was with him to enjoy this most emotional of farewells.[44]

He continued in private practice in gastroenterology in his Newtown rooms for two more years. When he finally decided to give up all medical practice at the age of seventy-nine, his intellect and energy were undiminished. He was planning a new career. He had applied to enrol at the University of Sydney again. And he wrote to one daughter indicating that he might just keep up a little medico-legal work using his elder brother's rooms![45]

Turning to the formation of GESA, there is no written record of who first proposed the idea of forming a society or association of gastroenterologists. However, it is clear that Stan Goulston was centrally involved. He had been in London for over two years, associating with and then working with gastroenterologists at Hammersmith Hospital. He would have been aware that a British Society of Gastroenterology[46] had been formed in 1937 and may well have been invited to attend one of its meetings. He had not yet travelled to the USA and probably knew little about the American Gastroenterology Association, which had been established in 1897.[47]

To what extent informal discussions had been taking place among Australian general physicians with an interest in gastroenterology about the desirability of a society is not known. The RACP, founded in 1938, now provided an annual national meeting at which these physicians could meet. They would have been aware that specialist bodies were emerging, as the Australian Association of Neurologists (formed in 1950), the Australian Cardiac Society (1952), the Australian Rheumatism Association (1956) and the Endocrine Society (1958) were already in existence.[48] Another venue for discussing the need for an association may have been the regular gatherings of physicians in Sydney on Saturday mornings at RPAH to discuss gastroenterology cases.[49] City-based groups have been the trigger for other specialist societies in Australia.[50]

The first known step towards forming an association of physicians interested in gastroenterology was a Sunday evening meeting held at Stan Goulston's Sydney home in June 1958. No minutes were kept, but Goulston when interviewed in 1992 had a good recollection of the attendees and of what was agreed.[51] The attendees included Dr Bill Morrow, Dr Bill King, Dr William Irwin, Dr Doug Piper, Dr Brian Billington and possibly Dr Ian Mackay. King and Mackay were based at the Royal Melbourne Hospital, while the others were based in Sydney. It is unlikely that King and Mackay would have travelled from Melbourne just for this meeting, so presumably it coincided with the meeting of the RACP held in Sydney in June of that year.[52]

Two decisions were made by the group. The first was that an inaugural meeting of a Gastroenterological Society[53] of Australia would be held in Adelaide in May the following year in conjunction with the annual meeting of the RACP. The second was that Dr Ian Wood would be invited to become the first president of the new society. However, while very supportive of the initiative, Dr Wood declined the invitation.[54] The first meeting, held at the University of Adelaide, was attended by twenty-five physicians and the attendees elected Sir William Morrow as the first president and Stan Goulston as one of six councillors. At a subsequent meeting, Stan Goulston was elected the society's first secretary.[55] The inaugural members of the society included those present in Adelaide and those physicians who had attended the meeting at Goulston's home the previous June.[56]

The convening of the 1958 meeting at Goulston's home, the choice of Goulston as the first secretary, and the following comment by the official historians of the society in the book written to celebrate the first fifty years of the society make it clear that Goulston was the driving force in getting the society established. Historians Russell and Sheedy wrote: 'Stanley Goulston from RPAH was particularly active in approaching interested individuals ahead of the meeting at his home'.[57] While people can readily mull over big ideas, in this instance the formation of a new national society of doctors, there has to be someone with the energy, enthusiasm and organisational skills to turn such an idea into a reality. Goulston throughout his life was extraordinarily modest and he never made such a claim but the record suggests that he himself did the most to have the new society formed. Support for this contention also lies in the observation that he was elected as the foundation Honorary Secretary, serving from 1959 to 1961.

Goulston then remained as a member of council for the following two years and in 1963 he succeeded Dr Bill King to become the third President. He remained a loyal and active member for the rest of his practising life and was a regular attender at the annual meetings. His status within GESA and beyond was confirmed in 1982 when he was elected one of the six Honorary Presidents of the World Gastroenterology Organisation,[58] effectively representing all the gastroenterology societies of the Asia–Pacific region.

If one adds to his thirty or so years as an Honorary Physician at RPAH the further years of clinical practice up until 1996, Goulston was witness to some remarkable developments in medicine, especially in his chosen fields of gastroenterology and hepatology where he led some of those developments, as will be seen in the next chapter. When he graduated in 1939, the main therapeutic drugs available were morphine, aspirin, digitalis and the first antibacterial, sulphanilamide. He was present at the commencement of the extensive use of the new technique of liver biopsy at Hammersmith Hospital. He saw the introduction of penicillin towards the end of World War II, streptomycin for tuberculosis in 1944, corticosteroids in the early 1950s, non-steroidal anti-inflammatories in 1960 and the introduction of effective oral diuretics. As well, he saw the discovery of Australia antigen – the cause of serum hepatitis or hepatitis B – in 1967 and the successful research that soon followed into hepatitis A and C.

Goulston began performing gastroscopy with a semi-rigid instrument and was able to change to the completely flexible fibre-optic gastroscopes towards the end of the 1960s, soon followed by their use in colonoscopy and then ERCP,[59] although he did not seek to be trained in the latter procedures. He must have marvelled when abdominal ultrasonography could at last detect gallstones and blocked bile ducts in jaundiced patients and when CT scans revolutionised the detection of myriad disorders.

Even as recently as the mid-1960s, he was using milk drips (into the stomach) to treat hospitalised patients with peptic ulcer. The advent of

H2 receptor antagonists in 1978 (cimetidine), the Australian research that uncovered the key role of *Helicobacter pylori* in the causation of peptic ulcer in 1982 and the marketing of proton pump inhibitors in 1988 (omeprazole) must have made a milk drip appear as if from a previous century. Indeed as a member and then chair of the Federal Government's Drug Evaluation Committee from 1967 to 1982 (see Chapter 11), he would have been more aware of advances in pharmacology than most doctors. All this and more happened during his years of practice.

CHAPTER 9

Clinical Researcher and Academic

Goulston was a very productive clinical researcher. For a physician of his era and one whose appointment to a major teaching hospital was as a visiting Honorary Physician[1] – a category of appointment without any expectation, responsibility or inducement to be involved in research – this was remarkable. In his career, he authored or co-authored over forty papers. In the current era, where some full-time medical academics claim publication numbers in the hundreds, this may not sound impressive. However, there were professors of medicine in Goulston's time with fewer publications. This was long before the era of 'publish or perish'. Many of Goulston's papers were published in leading medical journals and one was published in the highly competitive *New England Journal of Medicine*. At that time, few Australian clinician researchers had shared this honour.

His first published paper, written shortly after he returned from Tobruk, was a detailed description of his regimental aid post at Fig Tree Hill on the perimeter of Tobruk. It appeared in the *Medical Journal of Australia* on Anzac Day, 1942.[2] In it, Goulston focused on the physical aspects of working in a large cave and on the range of medical problems that he and his team dealt with, as well as the steps required to prevent dysentery and other diseases. His prose was precise but understated, as there was no hint of the daily dangers faced by himself and his battalion.

In the months before his paper appeared, little such information about the war was being published in the *Medical Journal of Australia*, although each weekly edition contained a segment of medical military news covering appointments, promotions, awards and casualties. In the next eighteen months, more articles relating to the war effort were published, especially a series of supplements on specific aspects of the best care of medical and surgical problems arising in warfare. These reports were issued by the Committee on the Survey of War Medicine of the National Health and Medical Research Council.[3]

Over these months, there were also several reports in the *Medical Journal of Australia* on war-related injuries and illnesses, but only two articles that could be compared to Goulston's enlightening and informative description of day-to-day medical life at the front. One was written by his brother Eric, about his secondment to medically assist Abyssinian guerrillas[4] fighting against their Italian colonial masters. The other was an insightful description of how different were the professional and ethical duties of a regimental medical officer when compared with his civilian medical officer counterpart.[5] Clinical reports from the war, none authored by Goulston, published during 1942 and 1943 included a method of improved localisation of shrapnel by X-ray,[6] bacillary dysentery in the Middle East,[7] relapsing fever in Tobruk,[8] war neuroses in Tobruk,[9] dyspepsia in soldiers,[10] anaesthesia in wartime[11] and desert sores.[12] In addition, reports were published of clinical meetings of Army doctors,[13] one of which in Palestine was attended by over 200 military service doctors. These meetings not only provided opportunities for sharing medical experiences and for continuing medical education, but also for comradeship in difficult circumstances.

Goulston did not write about his frontline experience again but in 1947, now back in Sydney, he wrote an article entitled 'The Need for a Medical Liaison Officer in Peace and War' for the *Medical Journal of Australia*.[14] This paper drew heavily on his experience as the Medical Liaison Officer for the Australian Army in London from 6 June 1944 (D-Day) until a year after the end of the war.[15] The paper demonstrated his interest in and knowledge of the history of how medical services helped to fight wars and how medical and surgical advances were often made because of the exigencies of war.

As already mentioned, towards the end of the war and its early aftermath, through the considerable range of local contacts that the liaison officer had developed, Goulston found himself helping to guide Australian medical graduates who had served in the Army to find training positions in the UK. Goulston ended his article with a suggestion that a similar role might be played in peace-time by a senior Australian doctor based in London who reported to 'a central medical authority in Australia'. If such an Australian central authority actually existed, his idea might have been taken up, but of course it never was.

In April 1947, not long after his return to Australia, he was invited to speak at a meeting of the New South Wales Branch of the British Medical Association.[16] He chose as his theme 'Recent Advances in Medicine in England' and his talk was subsequently published in the *Medical Journal of Australia* in July.[17] In his opening remarks he stated that 'he thought it best to talk of work done by men[18] with whom I had personal contact in London and in particular at the British Postgraduate School of Medicine'.[19] The first half of his talk focused on advances in gastroenterology and liver disease, and the second half on cardiac disease and the management of shock. Impressively, he had indeed spent time with leaders (Sir Francis Avery-Jones,[20] Professor George Pickering[21] and Professor John McMichael[22]) and future leaders (Dr Sheila Sherlock[23]) in their respective fields in the UK.

There was then a lull in his writing, presumably because he was fully engaged in establishing his own medical practice as a consultant physician, helping to establish gastroenterology as an independent specialist service at the Royal Prince Alfred Hospital (see Chapter 8) and adjusting to being back at home with his wife to raise a young family. His first paper based on clinical cases that he was now seeing in Sydney was published in September 1951[24] as the leading article in the *Medical Journal of Australia.* This described two patients observed over a number of years at Concord Repatriation Hospital in Sydney with 'cholangiolitic hepatitis', a then poorly understood cause of jaundice. Valuable because both patients had been investigated with percutaneous liver biopsies, then a new technique, the two cases probably did not advance current knowledge. However, this type of liver disease[25] was to become a research focus of the team that Morrow and Goulston were steadily building at RPAH.

Between 1952 and 1956, he was an energetic contributor to the Australian medical literature, publishing papers on infectious hepatitis,[26] the treatment of peptic ulcer,[27] the management of hiatus hernia,[28] and the uses and limitations of X-ray examination of the gallbladder.[29] In most instances, these papers were based on presentations which he had made to meetings of physicians, surgeons or radiologists, indicating that he was in popular demand as a speaker knowledgeable across the entire range of gastroenterology. His paper on the management of hiatus hernia, written for a surgical readership, was provocative but also objective and based on evidence. He had examined the records of a large series of patients who had undergone surgery for hiatus hernia at RPAH between 1951 and 1955 and had personally reviewed two-thirds of the patients. He found that overall, the results of surgery were poor and he advised against surgery, other than for patients with complications of hernias. By 'complications' he meant stricture, bleeding, obstruction and severe pain. He also advocated for a larger role for physicians in the care of these patients. He was ahead of his time with his observations, because as better tests were introduced – including fibre-optic endoscopy and measurement of the pressure in the lower oesophageal sphincter (valve) – it gradually became accepted that the underlying pathology was not the hiatus hernia but a defective sphincter. The focus of the surgeons slowly changed in step with these emerging observations.

Goulston's 1953 paper in the *Medical Journal of Australia* on infectious hepatitis was a *tour de force*, not only for the effort he had put into documenting the course of this disease in eighty-three patients admitted to the RPAH between 1949 and 1951 and followed until 1953, but also for the depth of his analysis and discussion. Here one can see the beginnings of sorting out acute hepatitis of viral origin from a similar presentation of an auto-immune inflammatory process in the liver. In the late 1960s, auto-immune liver disease became a research focus of the Gastroenterology Unit (GE Unit),[30] a research interest shared with the Clinical Research

Unit (CRU) at RPAH headed initially by Dr Ruthven Blackburn.[31] Soon a competitive research rivalry developed between the GE Unit at RPAH and the Clinical Research Unit at the Royal Melbourne Hospital, now headed by Dr Ian Mackay.

Dr Blackburn had also served in the Army, rising to the level of Lieutenant Colonel and Commanding Officer of the Army's Medical Research Unit in Cairns, where important research was undertaken to help prevent malaria[32] in Australian troops fighting against the Japanese. Like Goulston, Blackburn was appointed to the RPAH after discharge from the Army. He took leave for a year of further training as a Rockefeller Foundation Fellow at Columbia University in New York. On his return, he was made Head of the new CRU. He was in a position to observe Goulston's academic bent and when Blackburn was made Professor of Medicine based at RPAH, he soon appointed Goulston as one of his three part-time lecturers.[33] Blackburn and Goulston became life-long friends.

As mentioned in the previous chapter, Goulston persuaded pathologist Dr Vincent McGovern to take a personal interest in gastrointestinal pathology, initially with biopsies of the liver, small intestine and rectum and later also with biopsies of the oesophagus, stomach and colon. This McGovern did and as a result became an international expert in the field and a leader in pathology in Australia.[34] McGovern agreed as well to regularly attend the weekly case discussion meetings held in the GE Unit, where he presented and discussed the pathology finding relating to each case.

Goulston and McGovern became firm friends and together undertook some ground-breaking clinical studies. Alike in temperament, as McGovern was also a humble, quiet-spoken man, they were different in other ways as McGovern was a devout Catholic and never married. The warmth of their relationship was evidenced in a beautiful tribute that Goulston wrote for the Australian pathology journal on the passing of his long-standing colleague.[35] Goulston's tribute also depicts the sacrifices that both men were making in the pursuit of new knowledge and understanding of the diseases which they were encountering. Much of their research was done after-hours and squeezed into a busy professional life – and, for Goulston, a busy family life.

McGovern was generous with his time. Not only did he put aside an hour a week to attend the case presentations in the GE Unit, but he accepted without demur when Goulston would arrive in the Pathology Department, medical students in tow, to discuss the pathology findings of patients in Goulston's general medical unit.[36]

Together they studied and reported on the then poorly understood diseases of the colon, Crohn's disease,[37] ischaemic colitis[38] and pseudomembranous colitis,[39] the last of which was shown in 1978 to be caused by a toxin released by the bacterium, *Clostridium difficile*. However, long before this was discovered, McGovern had predicted, as early as 1965 and based solely on what he had seen under the microscope, that the changes would eventually be shown to be due to a toxin.[40]

Their most important and novel discovery – a finding that resulted in the paper published in the *New England Journal of Medicine* in 1969[41] – was on the nature of benign (non-cancerous) strictures of the colon in patients suffering ulcerative colitis. Up until they reported their careful microscopic examination of operative tissue removed from nineteen patients with long-standing ulcerative colitis and benign stricture of the colon, there had been a general consensus that such narrowing of the bowel was due to fibrosis secondary to persistent inflammation of the bowel wall. They were able to show that this concept was wrong and that the narrowing was due to thickening and contracture of a layer of the smooth muscle within the bowel wall. Their findings were of sufficient importance for the editor to commission a commentary in the same issue of the journal from pathologist, Professor Basil Morson of London, who was regarded as the world expert on such matters.[42]

Goulston and McGovern also collaborated to write a small textbook entitled *Fundamentals of Colitis*, published in 1981.[43] It is still available today as an e-book. It was an unusual book, as clinicians and pathologists rarely collaborated in this manner. It covered all known causes of colitis (inflammation of the colon and rectum), including the infectious causes as well as ulcerative colitis and Crohn's disease of the colon and less common entities such as ischaemic colitis and radiation proctitis. Pathologist McGovern made a large contribution, as the text explained in detail what was to be expected under the microscope. The book was well laid out and the writing was clear and succinct. The book was handsomely illustrated with radiological images, microscopic sections and pathology specimens. What might surprise a modern gastroenterologist is the absence of endoscopic images. This is due to the reluctance in the early days of colonoscopy to use the instrument in patients with acute colitis for fear of damaging the bowel or worsening the condition either in preparation for or during the procedure.

At the time the book was written, the authors had been studying cases of colitis together for thirty years at the largest hospital in Australia. They provided some references and recommended readings but, given their depth of experience, these were largely redundant. What came through most strongly early in the book were the insights of Goulston, the clinician. The message in the Introduction, wherein he emphasised the centrality of taking a detailed history and the closely related theme of taking steps to exclude treatable infectious causes of colitis, remains pertinent today. Later in the Introduction he emphasised the management of the whole patient with the chronic illness of ulcerative colitis or Crohn's disease, in the following words:

> The management of chronic inflammatory bowel disease, described in the chapters on ulcerative colitis and Crohn's disease, may cover a patient's lifetime and requires a knowledge of the clinical vagaries and problems that may arise. Due attention must always be paid to the patient as a whole, the personality, environment, emotional background, interaction with family, tension factors and the effects of medication. In no disorder is the patient/doctor relationship more important and mutual trust more essential.

This message similarly remains relevant today.

Sadly Dr McGovern died in a car accident in 1983, at the age of sixty-eight, so there was never a second edition.

By the mid-point of his career at RPAH, Goulston was recognised beyond Australia for his research endeavours, his publications and the quality of the work undertaken with collaborators, so it was probably no surprise that the editor of the London-based *Postgraduate Medical Journal* approached him in 1969 with a special task. The monthly journal was planning to devote its entire April 1970 issue to aspects of medical progress in Australia, timed to coincide with the bicentenary of Captain James Cook's arrival on the east coast of the island continent in April 1770. Gastroenterology had been selected along with cardiology, neurology, thoracic medicine and immunology for special attention. Goulston was among several well-known Australian academics who were invited to contribute, including Professor Ruthven Blackburn and Professor Ralph Blackett. When the issue appeared, its opening article had been written by Sir Ian Wood. Wood wrote of the contributions to immunology of Sir Frank McFarlane Burnet and linked Captain James Cook with Burnet by pointing out that both had been recipients of the Copley Medal of the Royal Society.[44] Goulston chose to cover the developments in gastroenterology in Australia over the years 1949–1969.[45]

During the 1960s, Morrow and Goulston now had the assistance of the first full-time staff specialist in gastroenterology, Dr Alan Skyring, who was appointed in 1960 with the strange title of 'Research Director'.[46] Together with a number of younger doctors (including Dr Brian Billington, Dr Jim Rankin, Dr Dick Boden and Dr Neil Gallagher) who had spent time in the unit for their training in gastroenterology, they were making careful observations about the course of an illness, fulminant (i.e., rapidly progressing) ulcerative colitis. In a series of reports,[47] they showed that the prognosis in such patients was dramatically improved by early surgical intervention. Through his quiet persuasion, Goulston was able to convince the general surgeons at RPAH that this special field was best left to one or two surgeons. Their work helped to change and vastly improve the management of this serious condition throughout Australia and beyond. A follow-up study twenty years later, co-authored by Goulston, confirmed the wisdom of this approach.[48]

The GE Unit's staff continued to take a deep interest in changes in the liver that they observed quite frequently in their patients with long-standing ulcerative colitis. Two early papers based on the endeavours of trainees Boden and Rankin were published in the *Lancet* in 1959.[49] Again these findings of Goulston, Morrow and their team were novel. They called what they saw 'pericholangitis',[50] now known as intrahepatic sclerosing cholangitis,[51] a serious concomitant of ulcerative colitis in some patients. With Goulston's encouragement, research in this field was a main focus of Dr Steven Mistilis when he was appointed as a full-time specialist to the unit in 1967 to replace Skyring, who had moved into private practice.

From the 1970s onwards, Goulston's focus and responsibilities shifted to include roles with the Royal Australasian College of Physicians and with an advisory committee to the Federal Health Department. In both instances, he found topics worthy of bringing to the attention of the medical community via scholarly articles.[52] He continued to write about a range of gastroenterological conditions.[53] After retiring from medical practice, he developed a new academic focus, as we shall see in a later chapter.

Sir William Morrow's name appropriately graces the RPAH Department of Gastroenterology, which he founded. However, Goulston's intellect, inquisitiveness, energy and academic inclination must have been a key to the rapid emergence of the department as the centre for gastroenterology in the nation. Goulston's academic and broader contributions were acknowledged by his alma mater, the University of Sydney, through the award of an honorary Doctor of Medicine degree in 1983.[54] At the conclusion of a long citation given by the Vice-Chancellor, he stated: 'Dr Goulston has been a consulting physician of high standing. He has also had a remarkable record in achieving constructive and important changes unobtrusively, most notably in the education of physicians.'[55]

CHAPTER 10

The Royal Australasian College of Physicians

The Royal Australasian College of Physicians (RACP) was established in 1938. Six years later, in early 1944, Stan Goulston sat and passed its entrance examination, becoming member number 159. By comparison, when Goulston took and passed the entrance examination of the Royal College of Physicians of London later in 1944, that college had been established for 426 years. As the RACP modelled itself on its London counterpart and as Goulston was to become deeply involved in the affairs of the Australasian college, a brief summary of the formation and early history of the RACP[1] will help to appreciate the roles that he played.

The first murmurings of a college of physicians for Australia arose early in the short life of the Association of Physicians of Australasia, which formed in 1930. This was a peculiar organisation as it restricted its membership to a maximum of seventy-five people. Although called 'Australasian', the association deemed its ten New Zealand members to be 'associate members'. Pathways then to becoming a consultant physician varied, but most physicians started their careers in general practice[2] and subsequently sought an additional qualification to enhance their status among their general practitioner colleagues. One source of such a qualification was to travel to the UK and sit the examinations of one of the UK colleges, as

Bill Morrow did. Another was to sit an examination for the postgraduate Doctor of Medicine degree offered by each of the four medical schools of Australia.[3]

Australian surgeons had already established their own college in 1927, the Royal Australasian College of Surgeons (RACS) based in Melbourne, so the consultant physicians were lagging. In 1931 the possibility of establishing a similar college for physicians was raised at a meeting of the council of the Association of Physicians, but it was not until 1935 that a subcommittee was formed to prepare firm proposals. These proposals were accepted at a general meeting of the association in May 1936 by a vote of 47 to 2. New Zealand physicians agreed that the new college was to be a joint effort, like that of the surgeons.

Now the problem was where the new college should be based. Canberra was still a rural town, so the only contenders were Sydney and Melbourne. After a short skirmish that included the Victorians harnessing an offer of support to the tune of £20,000 courtesy of the Nicholas brothers, marketers of 'Aspro', the Melbourne bid was gracefully withdrawn. That bid had helped to stimulate an offer of £25,000 from the New South Wales Government. Things moved quickly, as by 16 April 1937 the association had purchased a property at 145 Macquarie Street in central Sydney, where the RACP remains today. Approaches were made via the appropriate channel to seek to use the prefix 'Royal' and this was soon granted. The Royal College of Physicians of London offered its wholehearted support.

On 29 April 1938, the last meeting of the Association of Physicians and the first meeting of the new RACP were held back to back at the RACS premises in Melbourne. The first President of the RACP was Sir Charles Bickerton Blackburn, the father of Ruthven, and also a physician at Royal Prince Alfred Hospital (RPAH) in Sydney. Three vice-presidents were elected, diplomatically drawn from New Zealand, Victoria and South Australia. In December of the same year, in the Great Hall of the University of Sydney, an inaugural ceremony was held. Among the dignitaries were Dr Morley Fletcher representing the Royal College of Physicians of London and Dr Noble Wiley Jones representing the American College of Physicians.

In its first four decades, thirteen senior physicians from RPAH held leadership positions in the RACP. Six of twenty presidents, all eight honorary secretaries, seven of eight honorary treasurers and four censors-in-chief came from the RPAH stable. Several of the RPAH physicians served in more than one role. This high representation partly reflects the fact that the RACP was located in Sydney, making involvement easier and more attractive to local physicians, and partly reflects the standing and quality of the RPAH physicians. As noted earlier, Sir William Morrow was a foundation member of the college and served as President from 1966 to 1968.

In 1954, Stan Goulston put his toe in the water of college affairs when he accepted the task of Publicity Officer. He served for three years. He then served three terms on the New South Wales State Committee of the RACP, first from 1956 to 1958, and again from 1960 to 1964, and 1966 to 1978. In 1960 he was elevated to Fellowship.

In 1961, Goulston was appointed a Censor[4] of the RACP, following in the footsteps of his mentor, Sir William Morrow. In 1970 he assumed the role of Censor-in-Chief, chairing the select committee[5] responsible for all aspects of the examinations, written and clinical, that determined entrance to membership of the college and by extension determined the standard of practice of internal medicine throughout Australia and New Zealand. Goulston's time as Censor-in-Chief was a period of revolutionary change in approaches to physician training and in the methods used for the written examinations. These changes could not take place quickly as there was a need for thorough planning and wide consultation.

Goulston's final year in as Censor-in-Chief was 1974, as he had been elected President of the RACP to serve for two years, from mid-1974 to mid-1976. As well, 1974 was the year when the major changes to the training and assessment of physicians commenced and Goulston was provided space in the *Medical Journal of Australia* for two articles to describe in detail the rationale for the changes, the planning and consultation needed, and the end product.[6] Current-day contributors can only gasp at the space the journal provided but the two publications allow us to see that Goulston was on top of the educational and statistical issues involved and that he was able to explain lucidly why these changes were necessary. Within the two papers, there are hints that Goulston was aware of potential problems ahead and even a suggestion that his heart was not completely in agreement with all the enormous changes he was leading.

The system that he and his co-workers were seeking to change had been copied from the UK and had been used by the RACP since its foundation in 1938. It had much in common with the traditional final-year examinations in medicine at Medical School. In brief, the system was made up of two three-hour written essay papers, one focused on basic sciences of medicine and the other on clinical medicine. Candidates who passed were entitled to progress to the clinical examination held a couple of months later.[7] The 'clinicals' involved three phases: a long case,[8] several short cases[9] and a segment where the candidate might be asked to interpret an X-ray film or an electrocardiograph tracing or to comment on a pathology specimen.

The clinical examinations were conducted by the college censors aided, as the number of candidates grew, by co-opted examiners. Different pairs of examiners tested the candidate in each of the three phases. The only prerequisite to sitting the membership examination was to have had a minimum of three years of clinical experience after graduation and to be recommended by two Fellows of the RACP. Passing the two phases of the examination led to the award of membership (MRACP). Fellowship (FRACP) came later when colleagues were able to attest that the applicant had worked in internal medicine as a consultant for an unspecified number of years.[10]

The problems with the two phases of the examination (written and clinical) that had been identified by research included large variations between examiners marking the essay questions and unacceptable variations also in the assessments made by the clinical examiners. The solution to the problem with essay questions was to move to multiple choice question examinations (MCQs) that were computer marked. This greatly reduced the workload of marking essay questions but generated the need for multiple committees to draft and validate the multiple choice questions. As Goulston carefully laid out in his article, the MCQ system allowed for sophisticated evaluation of the capacity of each question to discriminate (or not) between candidates. There remained a dilemma of how to set a 'pass mark', which Goulston brushed over.[11] The dilemma has never been fully resolved. The MCQ approach could also be used to test a candidate's ability to interpret the findings of a range of investigations. Thus the third phase of the existing clinical examination could be omitted.

The problem of variations between the assessments of clinical examiners and the possibility that extraneous factors might be brought to bear in those assessments were barely addressed in the proposed changes. The reality of these variations was acknowledged but the general belief in Australia that observing candidates perform with patients was critical to assessment meant that the RACP was reluctant to follow the US decision to forgo such an approach in favour of supervisor reports. The college a little while later did take two small steps to strive to improve the fairness of the clinical examination for candidates. A system of 'calibration exercises' was introduced, which all examiners were obliged to attend. Here in pairs, they marked the performance of a video-recorded mock examination and the marks were publicly announced. Outliers were asked to explain why their mark was awarded. An evaluation of these exercises was never made. Several years later, in recognition of the problems, the system was altered again, now to provide exposure to more cases and more pairs of examiners.

The second step taken in Goulston's time was to use a method of a 'last gasp' assessment of borderline candidates. At the end of each day of examining, the censors (but not the co-opted examiners) met as a group to collate all the marks and discuss borderline performers. For any such candidate, the censor who had led the examining pair for the long case, and the second censor for the short cases, had to explain and justify the mark given. In anticipation of these discussions, examiners were encouraged in their marking to indicate whether the candidate was just at or just above the level of the mark awarded. This led to the strange terminology of 'seven with a lift' – seven being the mark that reflected an adequate performance and the 'lift' meaning that should the candidate perform less well in the eyes of the second pair of examiners, then the first pair (or the censor on behalf of the pair) would be prepared to argue that the candidate be awarded an overall pass. This system survived for many years but was done away with when the number of cases seen, and the number of examining pairs used, doubled.

Originally, entrance to the examination needed only three years of clinical experience after graduation. However, this was to change and result in the most far-reaching overhaul introduced by the RACP during Goulston's term as Censor-in-Chief. First, to be eligible to sit the college examination, candidates had to fulfil strict criteria of working under supervision for two years (after the intern year) in suitable rotations in hospitals and those hospitals needed to be accredited by the college for that purpose. Accreditation was based around aspects including the adequacy of the hospital library and the hospital's weekly education programmes, and the designation of a supervisor of physician training. Second, on passing the new examination, now called the 'FRACP Part 1', successful candidates were allowed entry into Part 2 training, to be called 'advanced training'. The latter was to be of three years' duration, during which a college committee would receive annual progress reports from supervisors (usually the head of a unit or department in which the trainee was employed as a registrar). At the completion of a satisfactory three years, there was to be no exit examination. The FRACP would be awarded based on those satisfactory reports. The MRACP was done away with. Introduced in 1974, the system described remains intact today, apart from the minor change in format of the clinical examination. Goulston and all those who worked so hard to plan and create the new system deserve much praise.

As part of these changes, the college also assumed a greater role in providing for career-long continuing medical education (CME) and assisting in the documentation of the involvement of its fellowship in CME. Many of the contentious issues around CME discussed by Goulston have still not been resolved satisfactorily nearly fifty years later.

As Goulston wrote in 1974, the changes to training and assessment

> basically altered the structure and purpose of the College from an institution concerned primarily with examinations

> and scientific meetings into one concerned basically with training, credentials, accreditation, and an educative process designed to maintain standards during progressive advancement of knowledge, and so enabling its Fellows to provide the best possible care to the public.[12]

In the acknowledgments at the close of his two papers, he paid tribute to the 'vast work' done by numerous Fellows of the RACP and especially to Dr Bryan Hudson, who had chaired the Committee on Physician Training and Hospital Accreditation.

Given the apparent success of the new training and examination scheme, what were the foreseen problems and for what reason did Goulston have reservations about the changes he was leading? He was concerned that the formalisation of the training of physicians might lead to 'an assembly line' production of a cadre of physicians lacking creative thought. He foresaw that assessment by supervisors in Part 2 of the training might be 'largely subjective and personal and could be potentially dangerous'. He lamented the lack of methods to assess non-cognitive components of a physician's capacity, such as attitudes and interpersonal relationships. Consistent with his personal philosophy, he wrote of failing 'to take into account artistic qualities, interest in the humanities, and knowledge of languages, which all contribute to the concept of the balanced, educated physician'.

Despite the work and travel involved, Goulston deeply enjoyed his years as an RACP censor. The group was cohesive and the members congenial. When Goulston was first appointed in 1961, the Censor-in-Chief was Dr Kenneth Noad and the group was quite small.[13] When Goulston left the group in 1974, there were eleven censors assisted by an additional thirty co-opted physician examiners.[14] Twice a year, the committee assembled for a week in one of Australia's state capital cities. By day, the work was demanding. A full day, usually a Sunday, was spent visiting each of the hospitals that would be hosting the clinical exams on one of the subsequent week days. All the volunteer patients ('long cases') who had agreed to assist were seen in detail by one of the censors with a co-examiner on the Sunday.

This system was also demanding of the patients, as each had to return for the day of the examination where one, two and sometimes three candidates would see the patient for an hour at a time. Over the subsequent two or three days, each censor was expected to accurately recall each patient last seen on Sunday whereas the candidate in front of him – censors at that time were invariably male – had just finished hearing the patient's story and examining the patient.

On the morning of each examining day at any hospital, the censors and their co-examiners were required to be at the hospital by 7 a.m. Their first task was to examine all the 'short cases' whom they would be presenting to candidates during the day.[15] In the examination, the throughput of candidates was intense as little time was allowed for discussing each candidate and the agreed mark before the next candidate was brought in. At the end of each day, the censors met to collate the marks and discuss borderline candidates. During the 1960s, all the candidates from each day were required to assemble late in the day outside the censor's meeting room so that borderline candidates could be called in for supplementary quizzing. Away from these days of examining, the censor-in-chief had the additional responsibility of handling complaints from failed candidates and overseeing arrangements for the next series of examinations.

These days of examining were tiring, all undertaken on an honorary basis. In the evenings, the group of censors would usually dine together. When the exams were held in Sydney, which was frequently, Stan and Jean Goulston would host the group at their home on one evening. Jean enjoyed entertaining. She had taken cooking lessons and looked forward to these nights. Her daughters assisted her in some of her tasks.

This was not the only hosting that Jean undertook on behalf of her husband. In the earliest days of the relatively small College of Physicians and the similarly small Gastroenterological Society, wives were expected to help organise the social programme whenever their home city was host to an annual scientific meeting. For Jean, this at times included taking wives of delegates to beautiful spots on Sydney Harbour. This was sixty years ago and such impositions on partners would not be accepted today.

In Goulston's time as Censor-in-Chief and as President of the RACP, the college made efforts to embrace physician training and assessment in Singapore, Kuala Lumpur and Hong Kong. Some young physicians from these three places had seen value in the qualification of MRACP and had travelled to Australia to sit the examinations, with variable success. To assist these young doctors, the RACP entered into reciprocal arrangements whereby trainees in those countries could pass a local written examination and then progress to the clinical examinations in Australia. In addition, for a few years the RACP took its clinical examination to these places with the censors of the RACP examining alongside local physicians. While this effort led to great goodwill for the RACP, it was eventually abandoned, partly because of the logistics involved and partly because each country developed its own approach. While it lasted, Goulston embraced the exchange wholeheartedly and made many friends.

In 1974 Goulston was elected President of the RACP, so he was required to step down as Censor-in-Chief. During his presidency (1974–1976), he was involved in some other important initiatives. As mentioned, in the preceding years the college had developed strong links with the physicians of Singapore.[16] Instead of their trainees coming to Australia to sit the MRACP examination, the college now took the examination to Singapore each year. The high point of the relationship came in 1974 when the college held its annual scientific meeting in Singapore. The Singapore Prime Minister, Dr Lee Kuan Yew, addressed the attendees and was made an Honorary Fellow of the RACP, with the honour bestowed on him by the college President, Dr Stan Goulston.

In 1975, after years of planning, hesitation, seeking of permits and a fund-raising appeal, extensive renovations and restoration of the heritage building at 145 Macquarie Street were commenced. By now the college owned the property next door, 147 Macquarie Street, so most of the staff moved into cramped conditions for the twelve months that the work took. Keeping up the morale and the work of the college staff during this difficult period was one of Goulston's responsibilities.

The hectic schedule of his presidency is reflected in his five days in

Canberra in May 1974. The first two days were occupied with a meeting of the college council, his first meeting as chair. The council held a dinner at which the Governor-General, Sir Paul Hasluck, was their guest. The next three days were for a scientific meeting of the college and during this time the president welcomed new fellows at an admission ceremony. Goulston had dinner on another evening with the Federal Minister of Health. He also had a meeting with Dr Sidney Sax,[17] chairman of the national Hospitals and Health Services Commission, where he learnt that funds had been provided to bring to Australia a Canadian expert, Dr Don Wilson – a friend to Goulston – to assist the RACP in planning for the enhanced continuing education of its fellows.

The president was expected to represent the RACP at meetings of sister colleges in other countries and this involved extensive travel. On one occasion, this led to his flying to London and back for a single meeting and he was away for only four days. Early in 1975 Goulston and his wife set off to Canada, the USA and the UK. In Canada, he attended a meeting of the sister college in Winnipeg, where he addressed the attendees on initiatives to share examination material between Canada, Australia, the UK and the USA.[18] In the USA, he met with the American Board of Internal Medicine to discuss the possibility of reciprocity arrangements in physician training. In the UK, he had meetings with their three Royal Colleges. In passing, he and Jean managed to spend a short time with their two daughters who were living in New York. There was no time to stay longer, since he was due back in Australia before attending the RACP annual scientific meeting and associated council meeting scheduled that year in Auckland, New Zealand. In 1976, he represented the RACP at a meeting of the American College of Physicians where he was granted the courtesy of an honorary fellowship.[19]

The RACP is named 'Australasian' because it is a joint college with New Zealand. Given the difference in populations of the two nations and the distance between our two countries, Australian physicians readily overlook their New Zealand 'cousins'. One of the responsibilities of any college president is to be sensitive to this relationship and the cultural differences between the two nations. During Goulston's two-year term as president, the RACP held an annual scientific meeting in Auckland. Goulston was up to the traditional Maori 'challenge'.[20] He handled this ceremonial 'challenge' greeting appropriately and endeared himself to New Zealanders by speaking in Maori at the opening ceremony.

Goulston had a long-standing interest in what is now termed 'professionalism' – the adherence of doctors to the values of the medical profession, which include such facets as altruism, respect and trustworthiness. He was alarmed from early on about the potential abuses by some doctors of the system whereby patients' fees were to be met in part or in whole by a national insurance scheme (first called Medibank and now Medicare). For example in the 1970s, when it was announced that reimbursement of general practitioner consultations were to be time-based, he wrote the following poem:

Time and Medicine
'Time is the moving image of eternity'
said Plato, with echoes from Judith Wright.
We live in a timeless land
Yet time governs our daily life.

'Time is money.'
The ten, fifteen and thirty minute consultations
Are suitably rewarded.
How long does it take to listen to the patient's narrative?
How long to examine?
To feel empathy?
To counsel?
To prescribe, legible or otherwise?
To fill in forms?
To record?

Time is precious.
Time to think, deliberate, reflect,
Time to identify with Nature,
Time to read, Time for music, culture, spiritual refreshment,
For family.

For proper doctoring time is not money.
Time for human values takes priority
To shape the patient–doctor relationship,
To complement the science and technology.

Many years later on a whim, he submitted this poem to the *Medical Journal of Australia* for its 1997 special Christmas edition. It was accepted and the editor wrote to inform him that it was short-listed as a potential prize-winner for the edition's best submission. As it was published without any commentary to explain that its premise related to a different era, its 1997 readers may not have understood his allusions.

Goulston held strong views about physicians misusing their position to exploit their patients or the national health insurance scheme when billing patients, so it was no surprise that he was asked to speak on this theme at a meeting of the RACP in Adelaide on 9 May 1984. His talk was entitled 'The Physician and Overservicing'. The full text was published shortly afterwards in the RACP magazine *Fellowship Affairs*, in September 1984. The paper covers events in the early 1980s when the Federal Government asked the Joint Parliamentary Committee of Public Accounts (PAC) to hold an inquiry into fraud and overservicing. In its report, the PAC stated that 'it had received evidence on the abuse by some doctors of the Health Insurance Act (Medicare), and has been shocked at the extent to which some members of this highly respected profession have gone to find ways of profiting from the system'. The evidence was of annual abuses totalling $100 million – the equivalent of $350 million in 2020 terms. In response, the government expanded its investigative staff and replaced its Medical

Services Committees of Inquiry with legally based Tribunals that had stronger powers. Heavy fines or even imprisonment were introduced for doctors who had patients sign blank Medicare claim forms.

As Goulston was not inclined to proselytise, it is difficult to discern his personal views in this paper. Perhaps they can be sensed by his quoting from a submission to a meeting of the PAC made by a group called the 'Rupert Public Interest Movement Inc.' which stated that 'medical fraud and overservicing is the creation of the medical profession and therefore their responsibility'. He also drew attention to selected areas of concern, including the overuse of endoscopic procedures, the excess use of laboratory tests by fellows of the college who were also approved pathology providers, and the dubious practice of physicians billing for daily post-operative visits for patients whom they had referred to surgical colleagues. He must have been distressed towards the end of his life to see that the overservicing issue had not been resolved and that a new problem of charging excessive fees had emerged.

The Neil Hamilton Fairley Medal is awarded by the RACP every five years and is the college's most prestigious and exclusive honour. First awarded in 1969, it is named after Sir Neil Hamilton Fairley who pioneered tropical medicine in Australia and made outstanding contributions to the health of Australian soldiers in both world wars. The medal celebrates 'world leading contributions to the field of medical science'. In 1984, Goulston was the fourth recipient. He had been preceded by Professor C.R.B. Blackburn (1979), Sir Ian Wood (1974) and Sir Edward Ford (1969). At the presentation of the medal, the then President, Professor Bryan Hudson, spoke in detail about Dr Goulston's contributions covering his Army service, his commitment to undergraduate and postgraduate teaching, his various roles for the RACP, his helping to found the Gastroenterological Society of Australia and his work chairing the Australian Drug Evaluation Committee.[21]

The RACP also honoured Goulston by commissioning his portrait, which hangs in the college buildings in Macquarie Street, Sydney. The portrait was painted by Judy Cassab, a renowned Australian artist who

Goulston knew (see also Chapter 6). Cassab was the first woman to win the Archibald Prize for portraiture and indeed won it twice. She was a versatile artist also known for her portrayal of outback Australian landscape.[22]

Later in his life, Goulston was distressed by decisions taken by the council of the RACP that led to the college enlarging its constituency by adding doctors from other areas of clinical practice as fellows. He felt that these groups – which included narrow fields such as occupational health, addiction medicine and sexual health medicine – were not sufficiently related to internal medicine to justify their inclusion. He fretted over the dilution of the sense of fellowship that the college should imbue in its membership. He was not alone in these views. Unhappy events involving governance issues at the college in recent years that have led to negative media coverage may well have been anticipated by him.[23]

CHAPTER 11

Other Service to the Community and the Medical Profession

In addition to the service which he gave to the Gastroenterological Society of Australia and the Royal Australasian College of Physicians, Goulston served on several other committees and organisations over his career that were related to medical education, patient safety or broader community needs. Soon after he arrived back from London at the end of World War II, he joined the Sydney branch of Legacy.[1]

Legacy is a charitable organisation established in 1923 by a group of returned soldiers from World War I who recognised that the more successful of their number had a duty to assist the less fortunate.[2] Under a national umbrella body (Legacy Australia Inc.), there are forty-eight individual Legacy divisions across Australia and one in London. Each division or club is responsible for providing assistance in its region. This includes financial assistance for the education of the children of Australian service people killed in active service. Legacy also provides financial assistance for other needs, as well as advice and support (personal, legal, general welfare) for widows and widowers of service people killed or severely disabled during military duty. Much of this support is handled via personal visits by Legacy volunteers, known as legatees. Most clubs also encourage social activities for widows and sponsor activities (e.g., camps and Outward Bound) for children. While some government support may come for specified projects, fund-raising is a continuous task for Legacy. The organisation is thus very dependent on public support. Its major fund-raising activity each year is Legacy Week, focused especially on Badge Day on the first Friday of September.

Goulston remained an active member for most of his life. In his early years, he served on the Medical Committee and on the Junior Legacy Committee. He later moved to the Mosman/ Lane Cove Division. In 1999, Sydney Legacy presented him with a certificate of fifty years of service.[3]

Goulston was proud of Legacy and the good work that it did. In his address to the New South Wales Jewish Ex-Servicemen and Women on Armistice Day 1985, he concluded his talk thus: 'How should we mourn the dead? Burke gives us the answer: "The true way to mourn the dead is to take care of the living who belong to them". That uniquely Australian organisation, Legacy, has done that for the last 50 years.'[4]

One of the medical bodies on which he served early in his career was the Postgraduate Committee in Medicine at the University of Sydney. He was on its Executive and Finance Committee from 1952 to 1956. The Postgraduate Committee in Medicine began life in 1932 under the auspices of the New South Wales Branch of the British Medical Association (now the Australian Medical Association) and in 1935 came under the umbrella of the University of Sydney. For several decades, it was the major provider of postgraduate medical education to doctors throughout New South Wales.[5]

A major commitment arose in 1967 when he was appointed a member of the Australian Drug Evaluation Committee (ADEC) of the Federal Department of Health. That year, his mentor and member of ADEC, Sir William Morrow, assumed chairmanship of the committee so it is likely that he recommended Goulston to the Health Department. Today the work of this committee (which since 2009 has a new name, the Advisory Committee on Prescription Medicines) is taken for granted by most doctors and is probably unknown to the wider community. It was first established in response to the thalidomide disaster, which came to light in 1961.

Thalidomide was a drug developed and marketed in 1957 by a German pharmaceutical company as a tranquilliser and an effective agent for nausea in the first three months of pregnancy. In 1961 two doctors, a paediatrician in Germany and an obstetrician in Australia (Dr William McBride), independently reported that the drug was highly likely to be the cause of a recent marked increase in severe abnormalities in newborns. The abnormality most commonly seen was a failure of limb development. The drug was withdrawn in Germany and Australia and, within eight months, the developmental abnormalities were no longer seen.[6]

This tragedy was a wake-up call that led to a much stricter system in Australia for the control and monitoring of the release of new therapeutic drugs for use in humans. At its centre was ADEC,[7] which began operations in June 1963 under the leadership of Dr Edgar Thomson.[8] Its task was to examine all the material submitted by pharmaceutical companies about new drugs and then to decide if there was sufficient evidence of efficacy and of safety to justify the marketing of a drug. Initially the committee was small and was made up predominantly of senior physicians. Over time, experts in various fields such as toxicology and basic and clinical pharmacology were added to the committee. A restructuring of the Health Department brought about a new section, the Therapeutic Goods Administration (TGA), to resource the committee with in-house expertise.

An early decision of ADEC was to recommend that a Registry of Adverse Reactions to Drugs be established and that clinicians be assisted and encouraged to report suspected adverse reactions to all drugs but to new drugs in particular. This was so successful that there was a need to set up a subcommittee, the Adverse Drug Reactions Committee, to handle the flow of reports. The database created is now the publicly searchable Database of Adverse Event Notifications on the website of the TGA.[9]

Goulston as a committee member served under Morrow's chairmanship from 1967 to 1975. When Morrow stepped down, Goulston was appointed chairman and served in this role until 1982. The committee met every two months in Canberra and ahead of every meeting members received bulky files of material to be read. In Goulston's time as chairman, ADEC considered around one hundred new applications per year. He took his task seriously and on his retirement it was noted that he had missed only two meetings out of a possible eighty-nine and none as chairman.[10] Considering that during his fourteen years of service on ADEC (1967–1982) he was equally committed to the Royal Australasian College of Physicians (1961–1976), this was impressive community service.

During Goulston's term as chairman, ADEC, acting outside its terms of reference, resolved a dilemma for Australian patients who might benefit from new anti-cancer drugs being trialled in the USA. There were regulatory obstacles in the USA that prevented Australian cancer specialists using new drugs in clinical trials with Australian patients. Goulston set up an *ad hoc* working party to examine the issues and was able to convince the Health Department to send the secretary of ADEC (a senior public servant) to Washington to see what might be done. The end result was that the US regulator allowed the sharing of vital information about drugs under evaluation, on a government-to-government basis. ADEC then established a representative working party to develop protocols for clinical trials with these drugs in Australia. The protocols made it clear that trials could only be conducted in hospitals and that the experimental drugs were to be kept in hospital pharmacies. This change has had lasting benefits; Australian oncologists are now world leaders in the evaluation of new drugs for cancer and Australian cancer patients have early access to those drugs via clinical trials.[11]

In 1978, Goulston accepted a different task and one that was not so onerous. A new monthly medical journal, *Medicine*, had been a success in the UK and the publisher now wanted to launch an Australian edition. The aim of the journal was to publish articles that summarised advances in all fields of internal medicine as a support for the continuing education of physicians. An honorary Australian editorial advisory committee was planned and Goulston was invited to be its inaugural chairman. The invitation arrived at a propitious time, as Goulston was about to finish his two-year stint as Immediate Past President of the RACP and so would finally leave the council of the college. The publisher was clearly seeking a highly respected and well-recognised Australian physician for this post and would have been happy with the result.

It was not long before Goulston was recognised in a much more meaningful manner, as on Queen's Birthday 1980 he was made a Member of the Order of Australia (AM) for services to medicine.[12] More honours were to come, for on Australia Day 1987 he was elevated in the Australian honours system to become an Officer of the Order of Australia (AO). The citation on this occasion was 'for service to medicine, particularly in the field of gastroenterology'.[13] This was a very popular award. He received over 230 letters of congratulation and each one was answered by hand.[14]

Late in his medical career, Goulston was invited to chair the Central Sydney Health Area Ethics Committee – a task which he accepted from 1988 to 1993. The prime role of the committee was to consider and, if deemed appropriate, approve written proposals for research involving patients at Royal Prince Alfred Hospital and seven other hospitals in the area. Much of the research involved clinical trials of new drugs, so he would have been well attuned to the potential risks to the research participants. Once again this was an honorary role and one that encompassed preparation by reading detailed research protocols and chairing long meetings of a group of health professionals and community members with whom he shared this responsibility.

CHAPTER 12

Poet, Teacher of Medical Humanities and Lover of Nature

From an early age, Goulston showed an interest in writing. He once said that he was writing poetry from the age of seven or eight. We saw in Chapter 2 that at the age of thirteen he had his first publication – not of poetry, but a letter to the junior section of the Sydney *Sun*. Five months later, now aged fourteen, he wrote this joyous letter to the same newspaper, with the title 'My New Dignity':[1]

> I've just had an exciting experience. I'm an uncle now – a real uncle. My sister has a baby. Everyone wanted it to be a boy, but it is a girl. However, she's very pretty and she's got a gold bangle on her tiny wrist. I held her in my arms before the father did – that was the experience. I was a bit scared I'd drop her, but I didn't. She's promised to be a Sunbeamer when she grows up, and win the Lady Denison Prize like Margaret Tait. The first thing she did was to yawn. By the way, she's got good lungs.
>
> It feels funny being an uncle. I've grown a beard, a moustache, and I'm only 14. Her father is a doctor, and I'm staying at the surgery while her mother is in hospital. You see,

> I'm very important.
>
> The trouble is, they can't find a name for her; at least, they have found hundreds, but can't decide which one to pick. She looks nicer every day, and I think I shall take her home tomorrow and keep her. Anyway I'm an uncle.
>
> Stanley Goulston (14), 6 Billyard Avenue, Elizabeth Bay.

Two months earlier, a piece describing his holiday joy of viewing glow worms had been published.[2] Around this time, he was also submitting poems to the junior pages of the Sydney *Sun* with some success.[3] In August 1930, his short piece entitled 'Seen in the Papers' was accepted.[4] It shows that from an early age he had a love of words and a sense of the ridiculous. It won for him a red certificate and read in part:

> News of the Weak – Doctor reports.
> Well Handled – The pump.
> A Singular Being – A bachelor.
> Light Work – The gas men's.
> How to Grow Fat – Breed pigs.

He also had a poem published in his school magazine in his last year at Sydney Grammar School.[5]

Many people try their hand at verse and doggerel, but few seek to write poetry and not all succeed. It is not readily clear why this is so but it has been said that poetry is a language within a language, and that in the language of poetry, the sound of words 'is raised to an importance equal to that of their meaning, and also equal to the importance of grammar'.[6] This idea about the sound of words is consistent with the observation that to enjoy poetry, you should read it aloud or have it read to you. Yet even when it is read to you, you may be disappointed; Goulston, from his experience of poetry readings, concluded that reading was an art and that only about one in six readers did it well.[7] The idea of listening and not reading silently is of course consistent with the manner in which one appreciates music.

Despite his failure to master the violin – a failure that to a certain extent worried him throughout his life – Goulston developed a love of music from early on. The family home was full of music and he had an extensive collection of records and later CDs. He attributed his appreciation and love of music in part to his violin teacher. Fortunately his love of music was shared with Jean, and many hours were spent together at recitals and concerts.[8] The Goulstons attended ABC Symphony Concerts regularly for forty years[9] and were early supporters of Musica Viva. He claimed the cello as his favourite instrument and wrote a poem bemoaning its fate at the hands of conductors.[10] He also loved the oboe. His favourite composers were Bach and Beethoven. He was never asked if he preferred poetry to music, but there is a hint of an answer in a poem written when he was twenty-one. In the poem entitled 'Music', he wrote:

> There is greatness in the art of books,
> And greater still the poet's art,
> The painter thinks his pot is full,
> And so did I until
> The speech of music kept me still.

Another indication of his deep interest in music came when he retired from clinical practice in 1994. He told daughter Diana of a plan to undertake a course in baroque music in the Music Department at the University of Sydney, but as we shall see he chose a different path.[11]

In addition, Goulston knew about words, having been an eager reader from childhood. He read widely throughout his life and even in his last years was still seeking books at his favourite bookshop or ordering books from the shop by telephone. And we have his Leaving Certificate result of a first-class honour to show that his talent for English was developed at a young age. His love of words extended to owning three thesauruses.[12] In addition to his love of words, he loved 'the feel of books'.

Writing poetry played a variable and changing role in his life but was never truly central to it; rather, it seemed to be a hobby to be used for various reasons, including to woo his future wife, to communicate with and show affection to his family, to mark and celebrate the life events of family members, to show his joy in his children and grandchildren (and keep in contact with them), and to reflect on the ageing process. We have seen earlier his love poem to Jean, written when he was twenty. Here are excerpts[13] of two poems written from overseas for Jean and of three poems written for other reasons:

Uncertainty (1940)
Can one seethe both with wonder and unrest
Seeing in one being all and none?
Can one feel desire coupled with perfect peace?
Can one both love and ignore in turn?
Can one behold in her all beauty
And next day find it gone

Tobruk Siege (1941)
To know I left you voluntarily,
Of my own free will. And that most eagerly
Out into adventure. Was I mad, insane?
Do flowers leave the sun and seek the snow?
And bees forsake the pollen?

Brooklyn in Winter (1978, for a grandson)
The ground below
Is white with snow
And it's a gray cold morn.

The car won't go
In all the snow
And stands there all forlorn.

Sixty Years of Married Bliss; for Eric and Nance (1994)
'Cheek to Cheek' and 'Night and Day'
'You are the One', there to stay.
Eric may have had his say
But Nance knew the game to play.

October 13, 1934.
Wed into the corridor
Of love for evermore.
What a stunning dress she wore!

Time and Old Age (1995)
Time, what improper haste
Propels him ever onward,
A built in accelerator
Hurrying him on,
He peers ahead, eyes on the horizon,
Plato's moving image
Towards Eternity.

He generally did not seek to publish his poems, with the notable exception of those published in the *Medical Journal of Australia* in 1970, 1993, 1995 and 1997.[14] In 2007, at the age of ninety-two, he published a small book of selected poems; the title, *Poetry for Pleasure*, is apt. Through this publication comes the image of a sensitive, wise, genial and loving family man and a 'thoroughly good bloke'.[15] The publication was not his idea; it was a project suggested and fostered by his caring nephew, Kerry Goulston, with the aim of giving Stan some joy and purpose in life after the death of Jean. The poems chosen came from a collection of hundreds.[16] Stan's good friend and colleague, Miles Little, wrote a beautiful Foreword to *Poetry for Pleasure* and, among many insightful comments, observed in particular that through all the book 'runs his love for his family and his fascination with words'.

In pursuit of this hobby, Stan did not allocate set times for planning and writing poems. In his own words, 'I don't sit down to write a poem, but something might happen and something comes into my mind and I might work on it. Generally when that happens the poem is already written almost. It's funny.' He rarely reworked a poem, but many were thrown away. Jean shared Stan's love of literature but not so much of poetry. Stan was never interested in 'studying and unpacking poems', as he found this 'a bit of a bore'. He did participate in poetry readings, so he was not writing in isolation. He was a good friend of Grace Perry,[17] a doctor recognised as a very talented poet; this was a friendship aided by the fact that Dr Perry was married to Dr Harry Kronenberg, who for many years was Head of the Haematology Department at the Royal Prince Alfred Hospital (RPAH).

Aside from his writing of poetry, he was interested in the poetry of others. He organised a poetry group that would meet at his home to present and discuss poems.[18] After his retirement from the RPAH, he established a most unusual event, an annual Poetry Grand Rounds[19] at the hospital, where he read selected poems and engaged the medical audience in a discussion of their relevance to medicine. Subsequently he accepted invitations to make similar presentations to other Sydney hospitals,[20] to a meeting of the New South Wales Society of the History of Medicine,[21] and to the University of the Third Age.

This concept may have been in his mind as long ago as 1960, when he wrote a poem entitled 'Hospital Grand Rounds'. In part, it read:

> Sitting in the audience I ponder
> How restore the patient's narrative
> The meaning of the illness
> Understanding of suffering
> The balance of science and wondering? …

> An appropriate literary resource
> To illuminate and illustrate
> Fundamental human problems?
> Prose and poetry renderings
> To supply and create a tour de force?

The first such Grand Rounds, entitled 'Medicine and Poetry', at RPAH in 1999 was exceptionally well attended. His brother Eric was present and soon after wrote excitedly to his niece, Stan's eldest daughter, about how well the event went. The selected poems had been printed and a copy given to all attendees. Eric declared that the chosen poems were 'beautifully rendered', there was good audience participation and that Stan had been invited to present Grand Rounds the following year. Eric concluded that 'you would have been proud of the reception given him'.[22]

Another senior doctor present observed:

> Then Stan began to read from modern poems expressing feelings of loss, despair, joy and reconciliation experienced by doctors as participants and bystanders in the drama of life. The discussion of the readings was fitful, emotions have little place in ordinary medical meetings, and a subdued audience dispersed afterwards to their afternoon tasks. Over weeks and months the impact of that session grew and further invitations to Stan to return to Grand Rounds followed. He has convinced many of the value of poetry in medicine.[23]

Miles Little, surgeon, friend to Goulston and a published poet, attended every year and recalled that the lecture theatre was always crowded. He found the occasions memorable and was taken by Goulston's quietly enunciated and articulated recitations, allowing the words of each poem to tell their own story.[24]

Goulston has left with his family the poems he selected for most of the events. For example, on Friday 12 October 2001 the poems selected and circulated included those of Peter Skrzynecki, Yehuda Amichal, John Wright, Peter Goldsworthy, Bruce Dawe, W.H. Auden, Federico Garcia Lorca, Seamus Heaney, Rumi, Michael Dransfield, Miroslav Holub and Wendy Cope. We don't know which poems he read and opened up for discussion on that day, as he usually only used five or so. Their themes included death, grief, cancer, suicide, drug addiction, compliance with medical advice, and leadership. Perhaps one can readily imagine the discussion that ensued from the following poem written by Dr John Wright in 1998, entitled 'Therapy':[25]

You attribute my recovery
to nor trip tyline –
its effect on neurotransmitters,
on the a myg dala.

You barely nod towards your worth –
insisting on blood levels,
on a therapeutic dose.

While I credit half our success
to the pear tree blossoming white
beyond your left shoulder,

to the wisteria –
its pink flowers hanging
lush and fragrant
over the portico,
to the warmth of your hand.

After giving up medical practice at the age of seventy-nine, Goulston made a remarkable decision: he would return to university to pursue his first love, English. He approached the English Department at the University of Sydney, where he was made welcome. He had a firm idea as to what he wished to study: believing that there was a close affiliation between literature as narrative and medicine as narrative,[26] he was keen to explore this link. After discussion with senior people in the department, it was agreed that he would enrol for a Master of Philosophy degree. Such a degree had been 'on their books' but Goulston was the first student to undertake it. He was also the first retired doctor to enrol with the English Department. His degree involved three years of work, including course work, a written examination and the writing of a thesis. In preparation for the course, he taught himself to type and became adept at using a computer.

He deeply enjoyed these three years of being a student again and experiencing afresh the intense interest in the comments on his submitted essays.[27] One essay was written as a response to the quotation 'All autobiography is fiction and most fiction is autobiography'. He used two works of Christina Stead to illustrate his points – an interesting choice of author, as in the opening paragraphs of his essay he establishes that Stead's mother died when she was two; her father remarried quickly and had six more children.

His course work included the study of early Australian colonial poets with nine fellow classmates. In another exercise, he was required to study one writer in depth and he chose Australian poet, Dr Grace Perry, whom as mentioned he knew through her husband, a medical specialist at RPAH. He readily passed the examinations set for him. For his Master of Philosophy thesis, his topic was 'Humanities in Medical Education: The Place of Literature'. As he explained to a journalist on the occasion of the award of his degree:

> Science is concerned with the disease, the diagnosis, treatment and possible cure, literature with the meaning of the illness to the patient. Literature develops our sympathies and makes us feel something of what it is like to be ill or to be the relative of someone who is ill. It can help us in coming to terms with the emotions and conflicts which are raised in anyone caring for those that are ill, bereaved, dying and grappling with the meaning of life.[28]

Goulston's thesis is an impressive tome of 280 A4 pages and covers a vast amount of research. It has three foci. The first is to mount the case for using literature to expose student doctors to aspects of medicine, illness and disease not captured in a science-based education. The second is to document, via personal contact with many academics, the extensive use of education in the humanities in medical schools in the USA and Canada and its almost complete absence in the UK (with notable exceptions in Scotland), Europe and Australia. The third focus is to select and annotate a range of Australian prose and poetry that could be used if or when such courses are introduced in Australia. A strength of this last focus is his appreciation of the ongoing crisis in the health of Indigenous Australians and his identification of a range of Aboriginal stories, plays and poems that could be used to promote discussion and understanding among medical students.

His thesis passed the tough scrutiny of the examiners. Some criticisms were made. Goulston as a mature student sensed that some of these may have reflected the personal interests of the examiners and yet 'overall he admired their observations'.[29] When he received his MPhil degree at a ceremony at the University of Sydney in 1997, it was fitting that he was presented it by the Chancellor, Dame Leonie Kramer, who among many roles was once the Professor of Australian Literature at the University of Sydney and the first female professor of English in Australia.[30]

His studies stimulated a closely related idea and he approached the Faculty of Medicine at the University of Sydney with the offer of establishing an elective subject for medical students on the theme of 'Literature as a catalyst in medical education'. His proposal[31] was readily embraced, particularly by Dr Jill Gordon who was Head of the Department of Medical Education of the faculty, and the option was offered for several years, beginning in 1998. It was open to first-year and second-year students in the graduate entry medical course. It proved to be popular with the students and was regularly oversubscribed. Goulston limited the numbers to around fifteen students to enable meaningful debate and engagement with all. When the group met, it was in a circle or semi-circle. The course ran for eight weeks. Each session was scheduled for ninety minutes but often went beyond that at the request of the students.

Through the course, he exposed the students to both classic and modern writers and went to pains to discuss not only the writings but also the writers and the situations in which they wrote. He prepared thoroughly. The students responded positively. Not only were they introduced to literature and its connections to medicine, but they learnt about the etiquette of debate and about verbalising a point of view in a secure and respectful environment. One student recalled being introduced to the works of Patrick White and the novels of Gabriel Garcia Marquez as well as to poetry. She observed that during the course, Goulston managed to touch on themes such as writing as an art form, medicine as a career, and suffering and empathy.[32] He also raised sensitive issues including Aboriginal health, and dignity in dying. While he usually provided his own interpretation of any piece of writing that he had set, he emphasised that there are never right answers to the questions posed by literature.

The collection of readings and poetry which he assembled for the session on Aboriginal health would have been challenging for a student with little or no knowledge of the true situation throughout most of Australia. The collection included a short table of health statistics, works of Indigenous poets, extracts from the first novel written by an Aboriginal Australian, and a short scene from the 1985 play of Jack Davis, *No Sugar*. Set in 1934, the play is about an Aboriginal family's fight for survival on a mission station. In the scene, the Chief Protector of Aborigines, Mr Neville, is visiting to celebrate Australia Day. The nun in charge of the mission welcomes the assembled Aboriginals with the following words: 'We gather together today to pledge our allegiance to the King and to celebrate the birth of our wonderful young country that we are so fortunate to be living in'. Soon she leads the singing of a hymn for which some of the Aboriginals have created a parody, which they sing loudly. Bedlam breaks out among the white participants. In the uproar, an Aboriginal man collapses.

The impact of this course is still recalled with heartfelt gratitude by a participant, now a specialist at RPAH, who attended as a first-year graduate entry medical student. At that time, she was unsure of her place in the medical course but felt reassured from Goulston's sessions that there is no single path to being a doctor. She felt privileged and fortunate as a new student to be exposed to an experienced doctor whom she found to be humble and inspiring, and whom she sensed to be 'a very special person'. Looking back, she could see that participation had a large impact on her subsequent career because she was helped to see the type of person and doctor that she wished to become.

Goulston received many letters and other gestures of appreciation, including a concert,[33] from his students. One wrote that he 'provided a gentle, dignified and incredibly compassionate and empathetic presence for us to aspire to'. Another wrote: 'my words cannot even begin to thank you for introducing me to the power of literature'.[34] When the opportunity arose, he used stories from his own wide clinical experience and exhorted his students 'to strive to be well-rounded, educated and inspirational human beings and doctors'.[35]

After three years of teaching the course, Goulston wrote a description of its rationale and content that was published in 2001 in the *Internal Medicine Journal* – a publication of the Royal Australasian College of Physicians. In his paper, he argued that Australian medical schools were lagging in the provision of teaching in medical humanities, defined as incorporating ethics, the history of medicine, philosophy and literature. His curriculum for 2000 covered 'the meaning of suffering', 'giving and receiving bad news', 'death and dying', 'the pros and cons of ageing', 'suicide', 'the role of narrative in medicine and literature', 'George Bernard Shaw's play *The Doctor's Dilemma*' and 'the historical study of bubonic plague through Boccaccio, Daniel Defoe, Pepys and Albert Camus'. His paper then demonstrated the manner in which he had used select literature to provoke discussion of the theme of death and dying. He concluded by stating that 'the addition of history, ethics and philosophy to literature would ensure that science and the medical humanities should be the natural collaborators in the education endeavour to produce good doctors'.[36]

Goulston was aware that the course he was conducting was not original, as he corresponded with physicians in the UK and North America who were teaching humanities in medical faculties before he approached the Dean of the Faculty of Medicine at Sydney University. He also acknowledged the early efforts of surgeon and Oxford arts graduate, Dr Tony Moore, at the University of Melbourne, who had run a similar course for five years in the 1970s,[37] stating that his course was based on Moore's ideas. Goulston deeply enjoyed this role, as he told his medical nephew, Kerry Goulston, that 'it was most satisfying thing I have ever done in my life'. His students were the beneficiaries of the rare combination of a very compassionate physician, a man with a profound love and understanding of literature, and a teacher with unusual ability to communicate with younger people.

He undoubtedly played a key role in bringing the study of literature into the medical course at Sydney University. Upon his retirement, his elective session was conducted for a while by Dr Jill Gordon, who also had an interest in literature. Dr Gordon was then able to have the university make a part-time, salaried appointment to the Faculty of Medicine of a staff member to teach Medical Narrative. Goulston's work had been honorary. The role of literature now forms a small element of the teaching component that also encompasses ethics and law.[38]

On the websites of other Australian medical schools in 2020, it is difficult to discern any formal teaching in medical humanities in the medical student curriculum, although there may be components hidden in the theme of 'professional and personal development' at some universities. As predicted forty years ago, one limiting factor for this aspect of medical education is likely to be the difficulty in finding people with the knowledge, skill and enthusiasm to teach in the medical humanities.[39] Stan Goulston would probably quietly remark that such an obstacle will never be overcome unless resources are put into the development of departments of medical humanities, as has happened in North America.

Goulston conducted the elective course for six years. He was pleased that one indirect outcome was the establishment of a postgraduate Masters degree in Medical Humanities at the University of Sydney,[40] which attracted twenty-four students in its first year.[41] In 2004, he gave up his role at the university, as he was no longer as physically active as he wished to be. Age was catching up with him. He lost confidence in his capacity to drive his car safely and he voluntarily relinquished his driving licence. His love of words and of reading was not diminished. He continued to do the daily crossword in the *Sydney Morning Herald* and he read avidly. Never one to rely on libraries, he said that he bought books by the 'armful' at his regular bookshop or telephoned the shop with his order. He stated that he read 'everything' but his favourite author remained Tolstoy.[42]

After music, books and literature, his other love was for gardening and nature. On retirement, he pondered taking a horticulture course at the Royal Botanical Gardens but could not fit this in. At every home he grew roses, for which Jean shared his passion. And for as long as he was physically able, he maintained a productive vegetable patch. But time was running out.

CHAPTER 13

Contemplations in the Third Age

Stan Goulston lived a long life. He seemed to have the capacity to observe the ageing process with equanimity and insight. He sensed that it was vital to keep using his intellect for as long as possible. He was aided in this by having the desire and energy to pursue his lifelong love of literature. Not only did he do this via the completion of a Master of Philosophy by thesis, he also applied his appreciation of the links between narrative and medicine in a practical manner by establishing an elective course on this theme for medical students. And he continued to write poetry. Through some of his later poems and via extended interviews recorded by his family for family use, when he was eighty-nine and ninety-three, one is able to appreciate how he reflected on his life.

First, his poetry of older age. At seventy-nine, when he gave up the practice of medicine and enrolled again at the University of Sydney, he seemed concerned that he might run out of time to complete the new task he had set himself, if the poem he wrote,' Time and Old Age', accurately reflects his feelings:

Time and Old Age

Time, what improper haste
Propels him ever onward,
A built-in accelerator

Hurrying him on,
He peers ahead, eyes on the horizon,
Plato's moving image
Towards eternity.
I cajole, threaten, entreat,
Slower, slower, slower
For my pleas and prayers he will have none.

Perhaps he was a little gloomy when he wrote that poem, for within a year or so his emphasis changed to be more optimistic and, in the poem 'Life after 80', he laid out a plan for maintaining physical and intellectual well-being. Here are the first lines of each of its two stanzas:

Life after 80
Maintain fitness
Walking is best
Keep reading and writing
Enjoy a good rest
Keep the brain active
With crosswords and bridge ...

Keep pace with grandchildren
Talk to the young,
Hear their wisdom roll
Off their tongue ...

When that poem was written, he had recently taught himself to type in preparation for his university studies and had become comfortable using a computer. His approach to learning to type was consistent with his belief that for successful ageing, 'the most important thing was to adapt'.

At the age of ninety, he was sensitive to how people might now view him and he expressed this somewhat joyfully in this short poem:

On Reaching Ninety

How should one behave at 90?
Brightly or lightly?
Loosely or tightly?
at 90
What should one say or wear?
What should one do or dare?
Would Rabbi Lawrence care?
at 90

And he asked what happens after the age of ninety in the first two verses of a poem entitled 'Life Continues after Ninety':

Living on after ninety,
Health reasonably maintained,
What is left to be achieved?
What still to be gained?

Now widower, children grown,
There still must be a purpose,
Still a debt to pay for all that happiness,
Than the simple label 'surplus'.

The extended interviews recorded in 2004 and 2008 provided Goulston with the opportunity to look back over his life. Several themes dominated his reflections. Most apparent was a sense of guilt, in that he felt he had been very lucky to be given opportunities allowed to few others and lucky to have had such a happy life. Linked to this sense of guilt was a feeling that it was wrong, even shameful, that he so deeply enjoyed his Army experiences. On one occasion he expressed this as: 'I still have that kind of feeling somewhere at the background that I don't deserve everything that I've got because in every part of my life I was happy, even in the war period'. Closely aligned to these reflections was the awareness of the debt that he owed to his wife, Jean, for her support for his long hours of work and his absences from home. He recognised that meeting all the commitments he took on during his medical career was 'tough on family life'. He was grateful to Jean, as she 'encouraged me in everything because I really wasn't home very much'. In the interviews he repeatedly expressed his lifelong sadness at never having known his birth mother.

There is nothing in Goulston's story to suggest that the absence of his mother prevented him from having a full life and a happy marriage, and, with Jean, raising a beautiful family. Yet deep down the absence of his mother gnawed at him all his life. It might be seen somehow as the equivalent of the suffering of an adopted child, but there is a difference as the adopted child can retain the hope of sometime finding her or his birth mother. Did this loss make Goulston a more empathic and caring physician, one who was prepared to spend time and effort seeking to understand his patients and appreciate how they coped with illness?

It is not easy to understand why he felt guilt over his enjoyment of his six years in the Army, unless it in some way reflected his sensitivity to the young lives lost. He told an interviewer, 'I was very lucky. I never had a scratch and neither did Eric.' It is a little easier to understand why he enjoyed his war experiences. As he looked back, he saw how much he benefited from mixing with other young men like himself, and some a little older, who came from all walks of life and all religions and none. He recognised that if his original expectation of being a junior doctor in a military hospital had come to pass, he 'would have been an ordinary bloke doing uninteresting things'. By being allocated to his own battalion, he saw the benefit of doing 'everything they did, and I got to know them well and later it became wonderful, a tremendous experience'. He must have had misgivings that as a young doctor, he was not going to fit in with his soldiers, but he found that those 'fears and so on were entirely misguided – it was the best thing that ever happened to me, it really was'. From other comments he made, it was clear that he was not forgetting or minimising what he went through, expressed as 'there were some very dark days and sometimes [we were] in areas where we didn't know what was going to happen'.

When asked why he enlisted in 1940, he emphasised that it was the expected thing to do and that 'everyone was joining up'. He was also cognisant that it was 'important that Jews pitched in'. He recalled that he was aware of what Hitler and Mussolini were aiming to achieve and that he had strong feelings about the rightness of the war, but these thoughts were not uppermost in his mind as a reason to enlist.

Like many returned servicemen, on coming home, Goulston's 'whole object was to forget about the war'.[1] And this he did, possibly helped by being able to immerse himself immediately in his work at the Royal Prince Alfred Hospital (RPAH). He did not join the Returned Services League, but forty years later he had a change of heart 'when society seemed interested in Anzac Day again'.[2] He began participating in the Anzac Day march in 1982. By 1996, the remaining numbers of his Pioneer Battalion were down to around seventy men. With another colleague, he led the Pioneers in the 2000 March. By 2004, only fifteen or fewer were there to participate. He was saddened as the numbers fell away but his sadness was tempered by his recognition that at their age, the deaths were 'physiological which is normal, anything that is physiological is good … just part of the ongoing stream of things'.

He found in later life that he deeply enjoyed meeting his wartime comrades and talking about the war. He welcomed Pioneer Battalion members to his home for parties and was pleased that Jean got to meet these men. His last Anzac Day march was in 2007, when he was ninety-two. Despite this reconnection with his battalion, he had no desire to return to Tobruk. When pressed, he declared 'I have no interest and don't want to go back there … it's all clear in my mind and I like it that way'.

He and Jean remained physically active well into old age. Good friend Miles Little recounted that when the Goulstons were in their eighties, he arrived home to find a message to call them. He phoned and received no answer. Fearing the worst, he drove to their home and was met by Jean coming off the tennis court and Stan coming down a ladder from the roof of their house! Jean insisted that he stay for lunch.

Stan kept in close contact with brother Eric. Eric lived to the age of 100, dying in 2006. For much of their lives there was telephone contact every day. Some of this may have been connected to their shared dabbling in the stock market. Stan also kept in regular contact with good friends, including doctors Maurice Joseph, Rowan Nicks and Ralph Reader. Stan and Jean were loyal to old and new friends, whether the friendships were made in Australia or on their travels. This extended to friends made in Japan and Canada.[3]

Jean experienced a major health scare in her sixties when she had a heart attack. Her condition worsened and she required urgent coronary artery bypass surgery. This must have been a difficult time for Stan, as he had to consent on her behalf to what was then experimental treatment. All went well and Jean enjoyed good health for a further twenty-five years.

In 2004, Jean became seriously ill and a decision was needed as to where she should be cared for. Stan insisted that she remain with him in their home and he devoted himself to her care for the next three months, assisted by his daughters. Jean died at home on 9 February 2005, in her eighty-eighth year. Stan's commitment to her care was captured by daughter Wendy when speaking after the minyan – the traditional Hebrew word for a quorum of ten Jewish adults required for certain religious obligations, but in a more modern sense, a prayer service – held in Jean's honour. Wendy said:

> I know she counted on Dad's loving presence through this last ordeal of their lives. His dear hands were on her head and hands constantly comforting her each day over the last months when his hands and voice could soothe her like nothing else. We supported his decision to keep her at home and avoid hospitalisation. He devoted himself entirely to her care and the maintenance of our household in her last illness. Seeing his tenderness with her and his staunch determination to ease her last days has been to me the epitome of love.[4]

Threaded throughout the family interviews were Stan's reflections on his happy marriage, which lasted sixty-five years. The couple had known each other for seventy-five years. He recalled 'wonderful times for most of our married life'. He admired Jean's even temperament; she 'was always the same, she was always right at the top'. He was able to admit there were 'times of quarrels and times when we had different views on things'. They shared a love of flowers and a love of music. In discussing the latter, he returned to his failure as young violinist but was grateful that the lessons had led him to appreciate and love music. One daughter recalls her father stating that if he had achieved anything in life, he owed it to Jean.[5]

It was after Jean's passing that Stan spent time selecting the poems for publication in the book, *Poetry for Pleasure.* He would have had little difficulty choosing his 1940 poem, simply entitled 'Jean', for it captures her essence and the depth of his love for her.

Reality, sincerity and beauty
    Are written on your face
Youth, freshness and health
    Are printed on your body.
Tenderness, friendship and courage
    Are written on your heart.

The thought and memory of your face
    Will linger till memory fails
To conjure you.
    The youth and freshness of your body
Will linger till that too
    Is dimmed.

But your heart with its calmness,
    Tenderness and feeling,
A curious mystery, both
    Hiding and revealing.

are drawn in part from that source and from more recent interviews. For one, her father was 'gentle and a gentleman – unusually gentle' and a compassionate man. Another appreciated him for being 'a very good listener'. A third described him to his face as 'generous and loving and being with you is a pleasure' but also regretted that when she was young, 'he was pretty absent' and that she 'longed always to have more time with Dad'. Fortunately this was compensated for as an adult, as her career in literature gave her a strong bond with her father. Shared among his daughters was a sense that at times 'medicine took all of his concentration and time'. However, they also recalled their father's good taste in selecting appropriate gifts for each daughter when he travelled abroad as well as his propensity at home to be an adept shopper who was prepared to buy the best quality items for them.[8]

They were aware of the sacrifices that their mother had made to support their father. One asked herself whether in their own careers and travels they 'were all fulfilling her fantasy [i.e., their mother's] of a fuller life'. They were admiring of Stan and Jean's marriage, one describing it as 'such an extraordinary relationship … the amount of pleasure and joy they got from each other is extraordinary'. Although two daughters were living abroad, all four women made sure that they visited their parents as often as possible and their father regularly in his later years.

While his daughters may at times have wanted more from their busy physician father, there was only joy in their recollections offered when the family came together in May 2000 to celebrate the sixtieth wedding anniversary of Jean and Stan. Diana spoke on behalf of her sisters in a beautifully crafted speech and Sadhana recited a poem she had written for the occasion. Diana was able to humorously cover, with obvious love and affection, her parents' happy marriage as well as their parents' foibles as perceived by the four daughters. The opening stanza of Sadhana's poem seemed to capture several aspects of Stan as father. It read:

> How many types of beans are there?
> you asked when we were kids.

broad, green, climbing, string – eagerly & glib.
But I sought out the trick
Oh, yes, Human Bean! That's it!

In his last years, Stan remained mentally active. He read avidly and, while he was able, he regularly visited his favourite bookshop in Glebe. As mentioned earlier, he described visiting the shop and coming out with 'armfuls'. He suffered a detached retina but retained good sight in the other eye, for which he was grateful. A friend took him to concerts frequently and a relative took him to see movies, followed by lunch and analysis of the movie.

His nephew Kerry Goulston, son of Eric, was also a frequent visitor. Stan had a special affinity with Kerry, who had followed his path into medicine and gastroenterology. Thus they had medicine and other interests in common, especially literature and plants. After Jean's passing and as his uncle aged, Kerry's warm support and camaraderie became crucial to Stan's well-being. Understanding Stan's longing to continue to be productive in some way, Kerry suggested the project of publishing the poetry book, helped Stan to select from hundreds of his poems, found the publisher, and nurtured the project to its completion in 2007. To the very end, Kerry was the steadfast, crucial anchor person that Stan turned to for reassurance and guidance.

There were still joys in Stan's life. At ninety-three, he wrote a poem about becoming a great-grandfather.[9] He attended grandson James' wedding in the USA in June 2005, where he joined in the dancing and then went with daughter Wendy to see the magnificent colours of the fall, staying in a cabin. In late 2008, he was keen to make the trip again for the wedding of a granddaughter in New York. He was sensitive to his family's resistance to the idea and reluctantly stayed home. In the background from the age of about eighty was the problem of a painful hip. This limited his mobility but he resolutely refused surgery and was reluctant to accept assistance.

At the age of ninety-three, now widowed, he admitted to becoming 'a bit despondent' but added that 'I have no right to be'. He experienced the loneliness of the end of a long marriage, missing Jean every day. In his words:

> Marriage is a funny thing. The more wonderful a marriage is, the harder it is when one of the pair dies. I think that must be the case. I never feel lonely for long but I miss Jean as much now as when she died, more I think still. I think of her at least sometime each day.

He described his despondency as 'physiological depression' and not an 'ailment' – a feeling lifted by visits and phone calls from his daughters, grandchildren, nephews and nieces, and grand-nephews and grand-nieces.

Interviewer Lucy Chipkin in 2008 posed the rhetorical question: 'It has been a very rich life, Stan'. In the modesty that never left him, Stan Goulston replied, 'I suppose so. I've been very fortunate really.'

Eventually he became frail and a little forgetful. His family employed part-time a woman friend of a cousin to assist him. They developed a great bond through a shared love of crosswords. She took him for walks in his wheelchair; he resented needing a wheelchair and he would have much preferred to have pushed it. With the aid of nurses and constant care from his daughters, he remained at home, as Jean had done, till the end.

Stanley Goulston, AO, MC, MBBS, MD (Hon.), MPhil, FRCP (Lond.), FRACP, FACP (Hon.), died at his home on 20 August 2011. He was ninety-six.

Epilogue

Stan Goulston's funeral was held at the Chevra Kadisha Chapel at Macquarie Park Cemetery, on 24 August 2011, and Rabbi Lawrence gave the eulogy.[1] His words were gracefully crafted and he spoke warmly and well but he was not in the best position to identify the legacies that Goulston has left behind, as many of these are medical. Others who wrote obituaries or letters of condolence to his family came closer with their accounts, but legacies can take time to become clear. Even this biography may have come too soon to identify all of them accurately. On the other hand, some were apparent during his lifetime.

It is abundantly clear that as a physician, he was a role model who inspired a generation of young doctors to seek to emulate his approach to patients, which was always courteous, empathic, patient and thorough. A contemporary physician and colleague at Royal Prince Alfred Hospital (RPAH) and at the Royal Australasian College of Physicians (RACP), Rick Mulhearn, wrote that Goulston was the 'image of kindness, tolerance, respect and loyalty'.[2] Good friend, physician Jim Lawrence, wrote to the Goulston family to say that he was a 'moulder of young physicians by example' and 'invariably generated trust, admiration and respect'.[3] Another good friend, surgeon Miles Little, commented that he was 'one of those people who would not fit the consultants' definition of a leader – not the charismatic type – he led totally by example'.[4]

It is also clear that Goulston had an extraordinary, although unobtrusive, impact on his chosen special field of medical practice, gastroenterology, at the RPAH and across Australia. At RPAH, he was a driving force in the foundation and subsequent growth of the first Department of Gastroenterology in the nation and for forty-four years served it loyally. He also drove the formation of the Gastroenterological Society of Australia (GESA). All current-day gastroenterologists who are members of the society are beneficiaries of his foresight.

There are patients today who benefit from his studies of, and insight into, a dreadful illness known as fulminant ulcerative colitis. He and his team at RPAH changed the often fatal course of this disease by recognising and promoting early surgical intervention – an approach now adopted worldwide.

At the RACP, the improvements to physician training that he encouraged and then helped to bed down are still in place nearly fifty years later.

One legacy yet to be appreciated or taken seriously by most medical educationalists in Australia is his identification of the need for modern, science-based medical practice to be leavened by humanity. Stressing the difference between treating symptoms and healing, and understanding how a doctor's relationship to a patient affects healing, he showed how doctors can develop their awareness of themselves and patients as people through the study of literature and poetry in the medical curriculum. He would be disappointed that still no steps have been taken to emulate Canadian and American medical educators in this regard.

Not addressed in any depth in this account of his life, Stan and Jean have left the wonderful legacy of four daughters whose successful lives they treasured and ten grandchildren who will ever remember their loving grandfather for his playful and poetic communications with them.

Never one to proselytise, Goulston was proud of his Jewishness and was faithful to Judaism. This was captured well by Rabbi Lawrence, who said 'we can truly say of Stan Goulston that he was a child of God. He was a man of good deeds; a man of action; a man of healing; he truly sought to improve the world within his expertise.' Perhaps lost in all this is Goulston's conduct during the siege of Tobruk. He was one of many heroes and is still honoured by Australian Jews. Thus he also left behind an example of which the Australian Jewish community can be very proud.

The inscription on Dr Stanley Goulston's grave depicts the man perfectly: 'Physician, Teacher, Poet. Greatly loved by everyone he touched.'

APPENDIX A

The Life of Dr Eric Goulston (brother of Stanley)

by Lise Mellor[1]

Eric Goulston pioneered a surgical procedure to relieve congenital tracheoesophageal fistula and become the inaugural Professor of Surgery at Haile Selassie University in Addis Ababa in the late 1960s.

Eric Goulston won an exhibition in medicine at the University of Sydney, graduating in 1928. His postgraduate study was broad, with residencies at Sydney Hospital, Prince Henry and the Children's Hospital, Camperdown, before travelling to London as a ship's doctor.

He spent two years at St John's Hospital, Lewisham, widening his surgical experience and obtaining the Fellowship of the Royal College of Surgeons of Ireland and later the Fellowship of the Royal Australasian College of Surgeons.

Eric's service in World War II was memorable. Married with two young children, he enlisted in the 2nd AIF [Australian Imperial Force] as a surgeon in the 2/5th Australian General Hospital (AGH), serving in the Middle East, Greece and Crete. Forced to retreat by the Germans, the hospital staff came under air attack in Greece and after the evacuation to Crete. They were eventually taken back to Alexandria by ship.

The 2/5th AGH was then moved to Asmara, in Eritrea. Eric was co-opted to act as sole medical officer to a patriot force of some 500 tribesmen under Major Shepherd, a former professor of English at Cairo University. This group was part of the Wingate base of Abyssinian guerrilla patriots in the south involved in a campaign to recapture Gondar from the Italians.

Eric's diary recalls the dates of the exercise: 8 November to 6 December 1941. He walked or rode mules through rough mountain country and after many adventures took part in the liberation of Gondar. For this work he was awarded the Gondar Cross personally by Haile Selassie. He then rejoined his unit, which was moved to Palestine.

When John Curtin brought troops back to Australia, Eric was transferred to the 2/11th Australian CCS [Casualty Clearing Station] and served in Papua New Guinea. His last post was as officer commanding the Australian hospital ship *Manunda*. When the Japanese surrendered, the *Manunda* was the first Australian ship to enter Singapore Harbour since 1941. Eric witnessed the formal surrender ceremony of the Japanese taken by Louis Mountbatten, then the ship brought back many wounded and sick Australians who had been Japanese prisoners of war.

Re-entering civilian life, he served as surgeon on the honorary staff of two University of Sydney teaching hospitals, Royal North Shore and the Royal Alexandria Hospital for Children, for thirty years. He pioneered an operation to relieve congenital tracheoesophageal fistula, a connection between the windpipe and the gullet at birth.

His skills covered all forms of surgery except neurosurgery; he was a relaxed, confident and very experienced operator who kept theatre sisters amused with stories and comments. He was a gifted teacher to generations of medical students at the University of Sydney and also developed a large private consultancy practice. In the late 1960s, when his distinguished public hospital surgical career ended at the age of sixty, he accepted the offer to become the inaugural Professor of Surgery at Haile Selassie University in Addis Ababa. Accompanied by his wife and daughter, he spent the next three years operating and teaching students there.

Ethiopian students, who had previously trained in Lebanon, were recalled and the medical school began producing a stream of intelligent and capable young doctors. At that time, the mix of feudal and modern society was fascinating: cattle had the right of way in traffic and the installation of parking meters was a dismal failure because of looting.

Eric revisited Addis Ababa fifteen years later to lecture. He found life there profoundly different, with a Marxist regime in power, media and mail censorship, restricted freedom of speech and movement, university leaders murdered and the royal family imprisoned without trial.

Eric retained a close interest in Ethiopian and Eritrean affairs. His last visit to the Asmara General Hospital was in May 1996, at the age of ninety, when he arranged for a young Eritrean surgeon to learn urological surgery at St Vincent's Hospital, Sydney. After leaving Addis Ababa, he joined an Australian civilian surgical team in Vietnam for six months, working at Bien Hoa, a hospital of 100 surgical beds, before returning home.

Each December for the next five years he managed surgical locums in Darwin, Alice Springs, Burnie, and Madang and Rabaul, Papua New Guinea. When his operating days ended, he acted as chief medical officer to the NSW Workers Compensation Commission from 1981 to 1990, and was also a medico-legal consultant.

He was the last survivor of his graduate medical year and the last member of the medical staff of the 2/5th Australian General Hospital. He regularly marched with his unit on Anzac Day; the last occasion was in 2002, when he was ninety-six.

To the end, Eric was an adventurer in spirit. Eric Goulston died in March 2006, three weeks after his 100th birthday.

APPENDIX B

'Humane Values in Medical Education: Shaping the Doctor – Literature'

by Stanley Goulston[1]

The 125 medical schools in the United States have established Departments of Medical Humanities, and over the period of the last 25 years Literature has featured in approximately one third of these with its own academic appointments.

In the United Kingdom, Literature and the Humanities in medical schools was virtually ignored until the General Medical Council in 1993 recommended in their publication, *Tomorrow's Doctors*, that medical schools include Special Study Modules in their curricula on subjects which could enlarge students' understanding of the 'wide range of cultural, environmental and ethical issues impinging on health problems'.[2] This inspired Professor Downie and his colleagues in Glasgow to draw up an imaginative integrated course 'An Introduction to Medicine and Literature', which in 1997 has been adopted into the medical curriculum by the Scottish Medical Schools of Glasgow, Aberdeen and Dundee. In Canadian medical schools also there are literary stirrings, especially at Dalhousie medical campus in Halifax where Professor T.J. Murray runs an enlightened extra-curricular program in literature, arts and sculpture. In Australasian medical schools there has been little interest in literature, with one inspirational exception in the 1970s by a surgeon, Anthony Moore, who single-handed for five years created a Medical Humanities course through literature in the University of Melbourne.[3]

The pioneer academics in the United States teaching literature and medicine in a medical setting emphasised that the study of literature was introduced into medical curricula not to provide culture or to remedy the omissions of premedical undergraduate study but to enrich a narrow curriculum that was focused, almost exclusively, on the value-neutral transfer of scientific fact.[4] Philosophy and Literature scholars have drawn particular attention to the essential differences between curing and healing, and between disease and illness.

What can literature teach medical students? What has literature to do with medicine? These questions echo the twentieth-century scientists who insist that science and medicine deal with the real world while literature deals with fiction, arguing that there is so much to learn in science and technology that medical students cannot afford the luxury of fiction and imagination. However, if science is real and factual, all the scientific facts are only shaped by the perceiver and are only partial. Further, much of what is accepted as scientifically valid today will be considered invalid in a few years' time. As Joanne Trautmann, the first full-time academic to teach literature to medical students, emphasises, 'fiction is said to represent the opposite of reality but fictional worlds are extraordinarily representative of the real world'.[5] We realise that the narrative of a story is a kind of illusion, but it is the illusion that is the vehicle of real experience of literature, and can help doctors to understand people and patients with similar experiences and points of view which may differ from their own.

It is interesting that at times fiction has preceded reality. In science fiction Frank Herbert's classic novel *Dune*, on which the film *Star Wars* and its successors were based, and the astronomer Fred Hoyle's *Fifth Planet* [co-written with his science-fiction writer son, Geoffrey Hoyle] preceded all space exploration, and Mary Shelley's *Frankenstein* and Aldous Huxley's

Brave New World preceded modern genetics, eugenics, in vitro fertilisation, embryo freezing and cloning. Also, the Russian nineteenth-century novelists illustrated principles of psychiatry prior to Freud and Jung, as seen in Dostoyevsky's *The Brothers Karamazov* and *Crime and Punishment*, and in Tolstoy's *The Kreutzer Sonata* and *Anna Karenina*.

Communication

Literature can help students in communication. Good adequate communication between patient and doctor is an essential need in medical practice and is a vital area in medical education. It is through communication that empathy can be established. Some doctors have considerable difficulty communicating with patients. Literature can teach students the use of words and the complexities of language portraying shades of truth with ambiguities and nuances of meaning, as do patients telling their histories to the doctor. Patients may use language and words both to communicate the truth and to obscure it. The same words, spoken by different people, can have different shades of meaning. For example, in Lewis Carroll's *Through the Looking Glass*, Humpty Dumpty's use of words to mean only what he wants them to mean raises the subject of words in dialogue, patients using their own vocabulary coloured by their upbringing and social environment. Again, in James Joyce's *Portrait of an Artist as a Young Man*, Stephen Dedalus talks to a priest. He exclaims 'How different are the words "home, "Christ", "ale", "master" on the priest's lips and on mine', differing in the sound, emphasis and force. Communication may often be non-verbal, expressed by signs, gestures or touch.

There is a wealth of literature illustrating all aspects of communication. To give one example of how literature can broaden students' view of communication I will quote a poem by Raymond Carver, celebrated American writer who died of lung cancer in 1988. This poem 'What the Doctor Said' was published a year after his death. It has been circulated in the abstract notes. There are no punctuation marks so the emphasis is my own.

He said it doesn't look good
he said it looks bad in fact real bad
he said I counted thirty two of them on one lung
before
I quit counting them
I said I'm glad I wouldn't want to know
about any more being there than that
he said are you a religious man do you kneel down
in forest groves and let yourself ask for help
when you come to a waterfall
mist blowing against your face and arms
do you stop and ask for understanding at those
moments
I said not yet but I intend to start today
he said I'm real sorry he said
I wish I had some other kind of news to give you
I said Amen and he said something else
I didn't catch and not knowing what else to do
and not wanting him to have to repeat it
and me to have to fully digest it
I just looked at him
for a minute and he looked back it was then
I jumped up and shook hands with this man who'd
just given me
something no one else on earth had ever given me
I may even have thanked him habit being so strong[6]

Students studying this poem may find the doctor quite brutally detached at first, and when he asks the patient whether he knelt down in forest groves, he could be sarcastic or empathic. There is ambiguity how the patient and the reader 'read' the doctor. When the patient just looks at the doctor and the doctor looks back, some deep understanding seems to occur between them. The poem pinpoints the shock, the limits and power of the doctor's words. The colloquial language and the different possible interpretations make this an ideal piece of literature for students to think about communication and how to tell bad news to a patient. Patients may be most helped by doctors who are capable of brief, intense moments of empathy so deep that it borders on fusion of minds and understanding.

This concept of empathy is identified by the American poet May Sarton in the last two lines of her poem, 'The Death of a Psychiatrist'.[7]

> Because he cared he heard; because he heard
> He lifted, shared, and healed without a word.

The gifted American physician writer-poet William Carlos Williams said of communication:

> Do we not see that we are inarticulate? That is what defeats us. It is our inability to communicate to another how we are locked within ourselves, unable to say the simplest thing of importance to one another ... The physician enjoys a wonderful opportunity actually to witness the words being born. Their actual colour and shapes are laid before him carrying their tiny burdens which he is privileged to take into his care with their unspoiled newness. He may see the difficulty with which they have been born and what they are destined to do. No one else is present but the speaker and ourselves, we have been the words' very parents. Nothing is more moving.

It has been scientifically documented that the drug placebo response can produce improvement in up to 50 per cent of patients, this response being real and measurable. Howard Brody emphasises that this placebo effect is matched by the patient–physician encounter, the measurable responses being neither imaginary nor fleeting. He uses the term 'symbolic healing'.[8] Anne Hawkins wrote 'In a time when quality of care seems to be overshadowed by issues of universal coverage and cost efficiency, it is well that physicians, medical students, and medical educators remember the importance of developing and cultivating this capacity – to communicate'.

Walter Benjamin describes the storyteller as the man who would let the wick of his life be consumed completely by the flame of his story. We are all storytellers and readers, doctors and patients. What we tell each other enhances or shrinks the humanity of each and deeply affects the degree of healing and quality of life for both.

Narrative

Narrative writing is an essential feature of medical practice and it is here that literature can have its greatest influence. The case history has all the qualities of a narrative or story. There is the patient's narrative and the doctor's interpretation and what he or she records. If the patient is referred on, the consultant's narrative will follow; if hospitalisation occurs there is the intern's narrative, continuation and nurses' notes; there may be the narrative of grand rounds, and finally, the discharge summary. During this process the patient's original narrative may be modified, submerged, radically altered or even lost altogether.

Some patients present their story as an artist would paint a picture, expansive, colourful, sometimes abstract, while the doctor, because of his training, prefers and writes a conservative, logical and orderly story. Doctors can better recognise the stories and needs of patients through narrative when they have developed their skills of reading with thoughtful interpretation, and when they appreciate the richness and joy of text. In history-taking, the danger is that the patient may be replaced by the disease as the subject of the doctor's narrative. A silent tug of war over the possession of the story may be the cause of tension.

The patient's story concerns 'the effects of illness in life'; the doctor's story concerns 'the identification and treatment of a disease'. The two stories are constructed from different points of view and this difference, essential to the care of the patient, is seldom acknowledged in medical school.[9] It is vital for the patient to feel that he or she has been listened to, that the patient is the enunciating subject. Several elements of the literary narrative contract – the art of writing, the frame of the narrative, the sequence, and the reader's response – heighten our sensitivity to how language plays a crucial role in diagnosis, treatment and healing. Learning to read and interpret literary texts develops skills analogous to those physicians use in their clinical narrative and diagnosis, and helps develop sympathetic understanding of patients as persons.

The relatively recent development of pathography, patients writing about their own illnesses, unites medicine and literature with communication and narrative. Pathography is a form of literature which could represent a reaction to the contemporary model dominated by the scientific emphasis on disease which may ignore the essential personal perception. Like science and crime fiction, it is now well established in its own right and includes notable writers such as Oliver Sachs, Lewis Thomas, Simone de Beauvoir and Anatole Broyard. Some patients have collaborated with their physicians in novels. Noted doctors themselves have written about their personal experiences of illness, such as the late Franz Ingelfinger, father of gastroenterology in the US and former editor of the *New England Journal of Medicine.*

Ethics

Robert Coles, noted American writer-psychiatrist, who teaches literature at Harvard to medical, divinity, law and education students argues that literature in medical education should emphasise ethics and focus on moral questions and decision-making.[10] There is a rich literary resource bearing on medical ethics illustrating and illuminating conflicts of ethical principles such as autonomy and justice, and highlighting medical research, informed consent, genetic disease and reproductive technology. Doctors as leading characters in classical literature provide exquisite studies of ethical behaviour as Lydgate in George Eliot's *Middlemarch*, Dick Diver in Scott Fitzgerald's *Tender Is the Night*, Sinclair Lewis's *Arrowsmith*, and our own

Henry Handel Richardson's *The Fortunes of Richard Mahony.*

Literature also increases the depth of understanding of fundamental life situations such as suffering, death and dying, problems of old age, childbirth, pregnancy, suicide, drug addiction and so on. For example, students discussing suffering in terms of the biblical figure of Job, Coleridge's '[The Rime of the] Ancient Mariner' and some of Chekhov's short stories should gain a deeper perspective of human suffering. The problem of drug addiction comes to life in the poems of Michael Dransfield, brilliant Australian poet who died at age 24.[11]

Literature also helps in the understanding of illness itself; what it means to be ill for the patient and family, as in Thomas Mann's *The Magic Mountain* (tuberculosis), Camus's *The Plague*, Kafka's *Metamorphosis*, Tolstoy's *The Death of Ivan Ilyich* and Paul Monette's *Borrowed Time* (AIDS).

Literature complements science in medicine. Science is concerned with the general, with patterns of disease; literature is concerned with the individual, the unique, the particular. Science is concerned with the disease, diagnosis, treatment and possible cure; literature is concerned with the meaning of the disease to the patient and those close to them. It can help with coming to terms with the emotions and conflicts that arise in those who are ill, bereaved, dying, or grappling with the meaning of life.

Quoting John Roy, McMaster University:

> Medicine protects life
> Literature interprets it.

Can literature change the understanding of non-literary people? Teaching literature to medical students does not ensure that they will become caring and compassionate doctors. But creating a literary atmosphere in tutorials dealing with communication, history-taking, medical ethics, and patient care could well develop a change of climate towards a definite interest in the medical humanities.

Rather than proposing a course of literature in the new postgraduate University of Sydney medical curriculum, I personally feel that literature could be introduced on the one hand into the 'Options' plan, while on the other, used in everyday teaching by educating the many tutors involved in the themes of 'Patient–Doctor', and 'Personal and Professional Development'.

A brilliant medical curriculum based solely on science and technology, which ignores the medical humanities, does so at its own peril. As Anthony Moore put it in 1978, 'It is my belief that if the art of medicine is allowed to weakly wander over a cliff, the science of medicine, with all its power, will not abolish gravity'.

In its statement of Aims, the Sydney Graduate Medical Program in 1997 declared its intent is to produce medical graduates who are committed to rational, compassionate health care and medical research of the highest quality. This is an interesting combination of aims emphasising the continual need for training in scientific research with an education towards a well-trained, compassionate doctor. I submit that use of a resource of literature including Australian and Aboriginal material can play a valuable part in this aim.

Notes

Preface

1 A. Sarzin, *University of Sydney News*, 7 August 1997, vol. 29, no. 17, p. 8.

1: Family Origins and Childhood

1 See https://www.geni.com/people/John-Goulston/6000000041370933612.

2 'Obituary, Mr Hyman Goulston', *Sydney Morning Herald*, 24 November 1930, p. 11.

3 The New Zealand gold rush began in 1864. The port was nearby to two areas where gold was discovered, Kumara and Ross. In 1867, Hokitika was recorded as the busiest port in New Zealand.

4 Hyman Goulston was married to Martha Solomon, with whom he had five children, John being the fourth born.

5 The exact year is unclear but Eric Goulston, Stan's elder brother, in a brief biography of his father written in 1977, claimed that John returned from New Zealand before his nineteenth birthday, which would mean that the family returned in 1888. See 'John Goulston (1869–1961) by Eric Goulston', copy held by Diana Goulston Robinson.

6 This was the Bank of New South Wales (now Westpac) in Bathurst Street, Maitland.

7 Stan Goulston, interview, 2004. Stan participated in lengthy interviews in 2004 and in 2008. The 2004 interview was conducted by his daughter Diana Goulston Robinson, assisted by her daughter Amelia. It was undertaken jointly with Stan's wife Jean and was directed primarily towards their childhood memories. The 2008 interviews, which took place after Jean's death, were conducted by Lucy Chipkin from the Sydney Jewish Museum on six separate occasions, and canvassed many aspects of Stan's life. All the interviews were recorded and later transcribed. Throughout this book, the interviews are referenced generally as 'Stan Goulston, interview, 2004' and 'Stan Goulston, interview, 2008'.

8 *New South Wales Government Gazette*, Friday 28 June 1895, no. 422, p. 4. In the language of the day, the business was described as 'drapers and clothiers'.

9 Brickfield Hill was a central part of the original business district of Sydney.

10 *Maitland Daily Mercury*, 13 April 1896, p. 2.

11 Stan Goulston was born on 26 July 1915 and his mother, Flora Goulston, died on 15 August 1915.

12 Sue Hallenstein (née Goulston), interview, 7 February 2020.

13 Eric Goulston to grandson Sam Goulston Robinson, letter, undated.

14 Golda Danglow came to Melbourne to replace her sister, Rose, as Jacob's housekeeper.

15 Golda Danglow was still living in Melbourne and the marriage took place at the St Kilda Synagogue.

16 This was supported by the recollections of Stan's four daughters.

17 Although now remembered as Rabbi Danglow, when he first arrived in Melbourne, his appointment was as minister to the Synagogue and it was to be some years before he was made a rabbi. See J.S. Levi, 'Danglow, Jacob (1880–1962)', *Australian Dictionary of Biography*, http://adb.anu.edu.au/biography/danglow-jacob-5878/text10001, published first in hardcopy 1981 (accessed online 11 May 2020).

18 J.S. Levi, *Rabbi Jacob Danglow: The Uncrowned Monarch of Australian Jews*, 1995. Rabbi Danglow died in 1962 and at his funeral he was described as the 'uncrowned monarch of Australian Jews'.

19 In an editorial in the Melbourne *Age* in 1957, Danglow was described as an 'inspiring tolerant humanitarian'. *Age*, 29 June 1957. See Levi, *Rabbi Jacob Danglow*, p. 283.

20 Stan Goulston, interview, 2008.

21 See https://www.geni.com/people/John-Goulston/6000000041370933612.

22 His illness was probably what in modern times would be diagnosed as 'depression' or 'major depressive disorder'.

23 Stan Goulston, interviews, 2004 and 2008.

24 Opened in 1878, the Great Synagogue is located in Elizabeth Street, Sydney.

25 New South Wales Board of Deputies, website: https://www.nswjbd.org/about-us/.

26 Raymond Apple, *The Great Synagogue: A History of Sydney's Big Shule*, 2008.

27 Ibid.

28 He made other relevant observations, especially regarding Saturday sport at his secondary school.

29 Sue Hallenstein, interview, 7 February 2020.

30 Golda's flexibility was attested to by granddaughter Diana. Interview, 2008.

31 Interview, 2008.

32 Stan Goulston described his father as 'very firm and very strict'. Interview, 2008.

33 Sue Hallenstein, interview, 7 February 2020.

34 That the proposed marriage would have seen his daughter relocate to America may have been a stronger influence in this. Wendy Goulston, interview, 2008.

35 'Those Who Serve', *The Hebrew Standard of Australasia* (Sydney, NSW: 1895–1953), Thursday 18 February 1943, p. 4. John Goulston's second daughter and

three sons enlisted in the Armed Forces. His second daughter Edna, a science graduate, attained the rank of Second Officer with the WRANS. Eric ended his career as a Lieutenant Colonel; Stan, as a Major; youngest son, Roy, as bombardier.

36 'Mr John Goulston's Visit Abroad', *The Hebrew Standard of Australasia*, Thursday 12 October 1939, p. 5.

37 Ibid.

38 'John Goulston (1869–1961) by Eric Goulston'.

39 The railwaymen's strike had paralysed New South Wales transport for many weeks. Sir Samuel Hordern later recalled 'how he and John Goulston had sat with two union representatives, three bottles of whiskey and a plentiful supply of cigars for three days' to resolve the dispute. *Sydney Telegraph*, Tuesday 13 December 1932.

40 See https://www.geni.com/people/John-Goulston/6000000041370933612.

41 Joseph Wolinski, 1872 – c. 1955. Wolinski's father had been a rabbi at Sydney's Great Synagogue. Wolinski painted landscapes and portraits and was a regular entrant in the Archibald Prize.

42 'Painting of Mr John Goulston', *The Hebrew Standard of Australasia*, Thursday 13 January 1949, p. 4.

43 Information provided by Kerry Goulston.

44 'John Goulston (1869–1961) by Eric Goulston'.

45 Kerry Goulston (Stan's nephew), interview, 25 March 2020.

46 Stan Goulston, interview, 2008.

47 Late in life, Stan described his stepmother as 'extraordinary … I think she did a wonderful job with us'. Interview, 2008.

48 In interview in 2008, Stan remarked: 'I stayed with her right throughout because I was very young but later on I became as it were older than she was, helping her and so on'.

49 The family had a cook and a maid, as did many middle-class families at that time. This common form of employment disappeared through the effects of World War II whereby women found better paid, less subservient and more meaningful work. This was also an era before supermarkets and many essential items were sold at the door of each home – bread, milk, green groceries, etc.

50 John Goulston travelled home from Circular Quay on a tram to the Glebe terminus and was regularly met by his dog as he walked to his home.

51 For a father not to accompany his family on a holiday sounds unusual now, but it was less so in the first part of the last century. Stan accompanied his stepmother and Peggy and Roy on holiday, travelling by train to stay in boarding house in places such as Katoomba or Mt Victoria.

52 Stan Goulston, interview, 2004.

53 Stan Goulston, interview, 2008.

54 The game involved placing a wooden stick across two glasses and breaking the stick with a sharp blow of the hand without breaking a glass. S. Goulston, 'Jolly Games Breaking the Stick', *Sun* (Sydney), Sunday 20 April 1930, p. 42.

55 Stan Goulston, interview, 2008.

56 Ibid.

57 Ibid. Stan often told his children that he had been a 'Glaxo' baby, referring to a brand of powdered milk with which he was fed.

58 Eric became a competent pianist while Olive chose to sing, serving in a mixed choir at the Great Synagogue for twenty-five years. Much to Stan's disgust, a new rabbi banned the mixed choir.

59 Stan Goulston, interview, 2008.

60 Stan Goulston, interview, 2004. Fritz Kreisler was a well-known, Austrian-born violinist and composer.

61 Ibid.

62 'A Tribute to John Goulston', *The Great Synagogue Congregational Journal*, November 1961, p. 5.

2: Youthful Years

1 Edgecliff Preparatory School was an independent preparatory school started by Miss Isabel Van Heuckelum. On her retirement in 1955, she encouraged Sydney Grammar School (SGS) to take over Edgecliff as many of her pupils went on to SGS. In 1956, Sydney Grammar School Edgecliff Preparatory School officially opened. Information provided by Ms Charlotte McColl, Archivist at SGS. See also https://en.wikipedia.org/wiki/Sydney_Grammar_School.

2 Goulston recognised that he had been treated differently. 'I was privileged. I went to Edgecliff Preparatory School and SGS – never went to a State School.' Interview, 2008.

3 Interview, 2008.

4 In an interview late in his life, Goulston remarked: '… and a little fellow aged 13 who just sung something and then does the Haftorah with the choir coming in – it was quite something. Looking back, it is quite a remarkable thing and also it gives you great confidence. Once you've done that, you have a different attitude to life. I found that was very helpful to my personality just to have done it.'

5 Goulston thought that the combined choir was of high quality and once stated that it was 'worth going to synagogue just to hear it. It was really a very, very good choir.' Interview, 2008.

6 Announcement: 'At Home', *The Hebrew Standard of Australasia*, 3 August 1928, p. 6.

7 See http://aagps.nsw.edu.au/about/history/.

8 Five of John Goulston's six children received a tertiary education – three doctors, a pharmacist and a scientist. Interview with John Goulston's grandson Kerry Goulston, 25 March 2020.

9 'School Notes', *The Sydneian*, 1929, no. 269, p. 21.

10 'Old Sydneians on Active Service', *The Sydenian*, 1946, no. 317, pp. 53–64. *The Sydenian* lists over 1,500 Old Collegians serving then in the Armed Forces as well as 72 Old Collegians who had been killed in the war. See https://www.sydgram.nsw.edu.au/files/the-sydneian/1940-1949/317_The_Sydneian_MAY_1946.pdf.

11 'Sydney Grammar School', *Sydney Morning Herald*, Saturday 14 December 1929, p. 22.

12 'School Training: Democracy and Education', *Sydney Morning Herald*, Saturday 13 December 1930, p. 15.

13 Stan Goulston, interview, 2004. In addition, *The Sydneian* reported that soon after leaving school, Goulston applied to join the Sydney Grammar Union – the school's Old Collegians association. Many years later, his support was also evidenced by a generous donation to the school's centenary appeal, as reported in *The Sydneian* in December 1957. 'The Centenary Fund', *The Sydneian*, 1957, no. 339, p. 107.

14 Some of Goulston's experiences at SGS can be traced via the school magazine, *The Sydneian*, which was described as 'a magazine edited by members of the school'. It was produced by senior students, closely supervised by teachers. The magazine also published short stories and poems from the boys. In that era, 2,500 copies were printed and were sold for one shilling each.

15 Goulston commented that in some sports and in some age groups, there could be up to fifteen teams. Interview, 2004.

16 In 1928 at SGS, Alan McGilvray batted in 23 innings for a total of 1,067 runs, an average of 56 and a highest score of 142. He also was a right-arm fast bowler and he took 44 wickets at an average of 13 runs per wicket. He furthermore bowled the most overs for the team. He later captained the New South Wales Cricket Team.

17 Stan Goulston, interview, 2004 and Raymond Apple, *The Great Synagogue: A History of Sydney's Big Shule*, 2008.

18 Herbert Webb (1850–1928) was a solicitor and past student who endowed this prize in 1901 so that a 'deserving boy, who has through no fault of his own missed taking a form prize, may have his industry rewarded'. It was valued at 10 shillings – the equivalent today of about $40. 'The Herbert Webb Prize', *The Sydneian*, 1924, no. 254, p. 42 and 'In Memoriam: Herbert Webb', *The Sydneian*, 1928, no. 266, p. 71.

19 The Intermediate Examination then was taken in Year Nine, two years before the Leaving Examination.

20 Stan Goulston, 'Talk Given to the NSW Jewish Ex-Servicemen and Women on Armistice Day, 1985'. Copy held by Diana Goulston Robinson.

21 Stan Goulston, interview, 2008. He recalled that he was ranked tenth in the state 'Order of Merit'.

22 Stan Goulston, 'At Watson's Bay', *The Sydneian*, 1932, no. 280, p. 32.

23 Eric's son, Kerry, believes that Eric chose to study medicine because of encouragement from Eric's father, John Goulston.

24 In an interview in 2008, Stan stated that his brother Eric 'influenced me in everything. I tried to copy him all the time' and 'I literally worshipped him'.

25 Reproduced with the permission of the Faculty of Medicine at the University of Sydney. See also http://sydney.edu.au/medicine/museum/mwmuseum/index.php/Goulston,_Eric.

26 There were many doctors in the extended family. One of John Goulston's sons-in-law was a doctor, as was a brother of one of the sons-in-law. Stan Goulston commented, 'we were surrounded by doctors and there was a very strong pressure to do medicine'. Interview, 2004.

27 Stan Goulston, interview, 2008.

28 Stan late in life stated: 'Jean's mother, May, was a fantastic woman. We got on very well together.'

29 It is of course incorrect to describe Jean and Stan as 'cousins'. The only Goulston cousins that Jean had were Roy and Peggy, the offspring of John Goulston's second marriage.

30 *University of Sydney Calendar*, 1939, p. 427. See http://calendararchive.usyd.edu.au/Calendar/1939/1939.pdf and *Sydney Morning Herald*, Thursday 22 December 1938, p. 5, https://trove.nla.gov.au/newspaper/article/17550990?searchTerm=university%20examinations.

31 Stan recalled that he was paid 17 shillings and sixpence a fortnight. If this is correct, it is equivalent today to about $80.

3: Joining the Army

1 The concept of Empire Day was to 'remind children that they formed part of the British Empire, and that they might think, with others in lands across the sea, what it meant to be sons and daughters of such a glorious Empire'. In 1958 it was replaced by Commonwealth Day, but this is not observed in Australia. See https://en.wikipedia.org/wiki/Commonwealth_Day.

2 One historian explains this drastic reduction on a government belief that a permanent professional army and navy were not needed. The 1922 Treaty of Washington may have also influenced government. Michael McKernan, *The Strength of a Nation: Six Years of Australians Fighting for the Nation and Defending the Homefront in WWII*, 2008.

3 Stan Goulston, interview, 2004.

4 Goulston enlisted at Paddington in Sydney on 1 January 1940.

5 As a result of his first attachment and subsequent postings, Goulston barely practised any clinical medicine for seven years. He thought that 'I was the only one that I know of who went through the whole of the war as a doctor never in a medical unit'.

6 McKernan, *The Strength of a Nation*, p. 12.

7 McKernan, *The Strength of a Nation*.

8 Robert Likeman, *The Thousand Doors: The Australian Doctors at War Series: Vol. Four: The Middle East and Far East 1929–42*, 2014, p. 12.

9 When Japan entered the war and their Army reached New Guinea (today's Papua New Guinea), the definition of 'overseas service' was amended such that soldiers conscripted to serve in the CMF only for the 'home defence' of Australia were now sent to New Guinea also. Graham Freudenberg, *Churchill and Australia*, 2008, p. 347.

10 Likeman, *The Thousand Doors*, p. 12.

11 Ibid.

12 P. Braithwaite, 'The Regimental Medical Officer', *Medical Journal of Australia*, 1943, vol. 1, pp. 137–142.

13 Every division and battalion of the 2nd AIF had the prefix '2' ahead of its number so that it would not be confused with the 1st AIF – hence the 2nd/1st Pioneer Battalion.

14 Gordon Osborn, *The Pioneers: Unit History of the 2nd/1st Australian Pioneer Battalion, Second AIF*, 1988, p. 180.

15 Jean and Stan announced their engagement on 29 February 1940 and celebrated it at a party at Stan's parents' home on that date, with Jean's parents present. It is not known if a wedding date was planned at that point.

16 To request a short period of leave to marry was not unusual for servicemen who had been made aware that an overseas posting was imminent.

17 Stan recalled that his future mother-in-law responded 'good heavens' and 'so wonderful' and 'right, we will have everything fixed up for Saturday and Rabbi Danglow will marry you in the St Kilda Synagogue'.

18 The announcements were in the *Age*, the *Argus* and the *Hebrew Times* and included details of the bridal party. Jean had three bridesmaids: Peggy Goulston, Mary Michaelis and Philippa Plottel. Roy Goulston was best man and Frank Danglow and Leo Slutzkin were groomsmen. Stan's brother Eric, already away with the Army, was unable to be present.

19 In 2004, Stan still warmly remembered Lucie Hallenstein's words. He also described his wedding as 'an absolutely perfect way to get married, no hassle, no bother, nothing'.

20 Zara Selby (née Kingston) was several years younger than Jean. Zara's parents attended the reception but Zara, still a school girl, was not invited. Later, Zara married Dr Tom Selby, a Sydney graduate, who had served in the Army and knew Eric Goulston well. When Zara moved to Sydney, she and Jean became firm friends, playing tennis together and attending concerts together with their husbands. Interview, 6 April 2020.

21 Jean was not alone, as already she had been befriended by the wives of other officers. As a group, they were known as 'camp followers'.

22 A speech Goulston gave at the Remembrance Night Dinner in Melbourne, on 22 November 1987, entitled 'A Doctor at War', gives this figure and the eventual battalion total of over 1,500 men. The speech was published in March 1988 in *Parade*, the official organ of the Australian Federation of Jewish Ex-Service Associations.

23 In 1940, the range of useful drugs was limited. Goulston noted that the only antibiotic he had was the new sulphonamide, Prontosil, and reflected that it had been invented by a German.

24 Osborn, *The Pioneers*, p. 179. It was usual for mothers, wives and girlfriends in Australia to organise a 'Comforts Fund' for the purpose of providing various items to a battalion.

25 Goulston, 'A Doctor at War'.

26 Ibid.

27 Ibid.

28 There is no record of how Goulston used this leave but it seems highly likely that he spent it in Sydney with his wife of four months.

29 Sue Hallestein (née Goulston), interview, 29 June 2020.

30 See https://commons.wikimedia.org/wiki/Category:Johan_de_Witt_(ship,_1920).

31 Osborn, *The Pioneers*, p. 179.

32 Ibid.

33 Goulston, 'A Doctor at War' and Osborn, *Pioneers*, p. 181.

34 Osborn, *The Pioneers*, p. 181.

35 Stan Goulston, interview, 2008.

36 'Aspro' was an Australian trade name for aspirin.

37 Osborn, *The Pioneers*, p. 181.

38 Goulston described being driven to Gaza to find the 'very senior' officer who was at a post-Christmas party. That officer acted at once. Goulston, 'A Doctor at War'.

39 Sue Hallenstein (née Goulston), interview, 7 January 2020.

40 Goulston gave the microscope to a young Italian doctor who spent some time visiting the A.W. Morrow Department of Gastroenterology at the Royal Prince Alfred Hospital in 1970, where Goulston was now the senior gastroenterologist. Osborn, *The Pioneers*, p. 181.

4: A Rat of Tobruk

1 The German Army marched into Paris on 23 June 1940.

2 Goulston wrote that the total population of troops at Tobruk was 35,307 before some were withdrawn. This was noted in a speech which Goulston gave at the Remembrance Night Dinner in Melbourne on 22 November 1987, entitled 'A Doctor at War', subsequently published in March 1988 in *Parade*, the official organ of the Australian Federation of Jewish Ex-Service Associations.

3 Goulston's total experience was his 1939 duties as a first-year resident medical officer and three months as a second-year resident medical officer, both at the Royal Prince Alfred Hospital in Sydney.

4 Many books have been written about the events in North Africa in World War II. The following are recommended: Chester Wilmot, *Tobruk 1941*, 1944; Chester Wilmot, *Tobruk 1941, Capture – Siege – Relief*, 1945; Peter FitzSimons, *Tobruk*, 2006; John Devine, *The Rats of Tobruk*, 1943; Alan Moorehead, *African Trilogy: The North African Campaign, 1940–43*, 1998.

5 S.J.M. Goulston, 'A Regimental Aid Post in Tobruk', *Medical Journal of Australia*, 1942, vol. 1, no. 17, pp. 494–496. In his 1987 talk, 'A Doctor at War', Goulston said, 'The enemies were the Germans, flies, fleas, heat, dust storms, boredom and inactivity'.

6 Gordon Osborn, *The Pioneers: Unit History of the 2nd/1st Australian Pioneer Battalion, Second AIF*, 1988, p. 183.

7 Stan Goulston, interview, 2004.

8 Goulston, 'A Doctor at War'.

9 Wilmot, *Tobruk 1941*.

10 FitzSimons, *Tobruk*; Moorehead, *African Trilogy: The North African Campaign, 1940–43*.

11 Goulston, 'A Regimental Aid Post in Tobruk'.

12 FitzSimons, *Tobruk*, p. 260.

13 Goulston, 'A Regimental Aid Post in Tobruk'.

14 Osborn, *The Pioneers*, p. 181. Goulston elsewhere wrote that he felt the Germans respected the Red Cross flag when it was displayed on a truck involved in bringing the wounded back from the front line.

15 Goulston felt that both aid posts were exposed. Unpublished paper by Goulston entitled 'The Figtree, the Libyan Campaign and the 2/1 Aust Pioneer Battalion', held by his family.

16 Osborn, *The Pioneers*, p. 181.

17 Goulston, 'A Doctor at War'.

18 One Imperial foot equals 30.5 cm.

19 His conduct is described in the citation for the Military Cross that he won that night. A copy of the citation is held by his daughter, Sue Hallenstein.

20 For a full description of this RAP and the work he did there, see Goulston's paper 'A Regimental Aid Post in Tobruk'.

21 Ibid.

22 Osborn, *The Pioneers*, p. 182.

23 S. Goulston, 'Talk Given to the NSW Jewish Ex-Servicemen and Women on Armistice Day, 1985', copy held by Diana Goulston Robinson.

24 Goulston described this event as follows: 'One night my CO [Commanding Officer] decided on a deeper than usual reconnaissance and wanted prisoners for questioning. I was asked to set up a forward aid post within enemy lines. My driver and I set out after dark in my one tonne truck called Aspro and were progressing slowly and well until the front wheel on the driver's side struck a mine. Most of the engine up to the dashboard was demolished. We decided to get out and walk back along our tracks. We did this and after slow progress were apprehended by sentries from a neighbouring battalion. Expecting to be severely reprimanded for our poor showing, when we eventually reached our HQ we were relieved that they were pleased to see us as they had anticipated we had been killed or taken prisoners.' Goulston, 'A Doctor at War'.

25 A granddaughter, Lucie Hallenstein, recalls being told by her grandfather that 'the whole front of the car just disappeared!!!' Interview, 2008.

26 His driver suffered perforated ear-drums and had to be evacuated to Alexandria. Stan Goulston, interview 2008 and Osborn, *The Pioneers*, p. 184.

27 Goulston, 'A Regimental Aid Post in Tobruk'.

28 C. Morlet, 'With the Australian Army Medical Corps in Two Sieges: Anzac and Tobruk', *Medical Journal of Australia*, 1943, vol. 2, pp. 221–224. The 4th Army General Hospital was fully equipped for major surgery and had X-ray and pathology services as well as a blood bank.

29 The Military Cross ranks just below the Victoria Cross and the Distinguished Service Order. See https://www.gov.uk/guidance/medals-campaigns-descriptions-and-eligibility.

30 A copy of the citation is held by his daughter, Sue Hallenstein.

31 Stan Goulston, interview, 2008.

32 'Vale – Dr Stan Goulston', *Pioneer News*, The Official Organ of 2/1 and 2/2 Pioneer Battalions Association, November 2011, p. 4.

33 Neil Gallagher, 'Morrow, Sir Arthur William (Bill) (1903–1977)', *Australian Dictionary of Biography*, http://adb.anu.edu.au/biography/morrow-sir-arthur-william-bill-11178/text19919, published first in hardcopy 2000.

34 One account has Joyce sneering at the troops as 'the rats of Tobruk – Germany's self-supporting prisoners'. *Pioneer News*, November 2011, p. 4.

35 Barlow was known as 'Lofty' because he was very tall. He was highly regarded for his skill and courage in defusing unexploded bombs. He wrote to relatives in Sydney that 'Lord Haw-Haw called us "Tobruk rats", so I thought I would make one of these medals for a joke. We presented it to Lieut.-Col. Brown, in charge of the Pioneers. So the fun began. Everyone from the General down wanted one of these medals. Men with many decorations made eager inquiries for this unofficial distinction. Since then requests have come from far and wide.' 'Rat Medal. Pride of Tobruk', *Cairns Post*, 8 January 1942. There may have been others who assisted in the design and making of the medals.

36 Sue Hallenstein (née Goulston), interview, 29 June 2020.

37 There were other informal medals created during the siege of Tobruk, as a circular medal was cast in dental plaster and around 300 were made. 'More on the Rats of Tobruk Medal', Numismatic Bibliomania Society e-newsletter, *The E-Sylum*, 2011, vol. 14, 17 April, article 14, https://www.coinbooks.org/esylum/.

38 Osborn, *The Pioneers*.

39 Excerpt of a report of the event from the Australian War Museum, copy held by Goulston's family.

40 '"Tobruk Rat" Medal', *Sydney Morning Herald*, Tuesday 30 December 1941.

41 'News and Notes of Old Sydneians', *The Sydneian*, 1942, no. 308, p. 62.

42 A surprise, as more than one historian has criticised Blamey for not visiting Tobruk during the siege.

43 'Vale – Dr Stan Goulston', p. 4.

44 Goulston earlier had been given by his engineering platoon an ashtray made from the propeller of a Messerschmitt plane that had been shot down at Tobruk, 'in appreciation of the work you have done for the Battalion'. Note addressed to 'Capt. Goulston 1941', held by Sue Hallenstein.

45 Goulston sent these home to Jean in September 1941 with a note to say 'These funny things are parts of captured Italian 2 inch mortar shells and were cut

down for me and stamped with the name of the garrison and can be used as egg cups. We can have them lacquered any colour we like. Pretty good eh – getting crockery from Iti's shells.'

46 Osborn, *The Pioneers*, p. 68: 'In the early days there was some dysentery but adherence to strict rules of sanitation under the watchful eyes of stretcher bearers in the company areas had overcome the problem.'

47 Ibid. The average weight loss of the battalion was two stone (12.7 kg). See also Peter FitzSimons' *Tobruk* at p. 434 for a fuller description of the medical officers' report on the state of health of the Australian troops by August 1941.

48 See https://en.wikipedia.org/wiki/Scipio_Africanus.

49 In addition to the two knitted pullovers, Stan received food parcels containing cake and tins of preserved fruit. Sue Hallenstein (née Goulston), interview, 29 June 2020.

50 In the siege, 776 Australians were killed in action and 2,112 were wounded. Goulston, 'A Doctor at War'.

51 Material prepared by Goulston as his contribution to the written history of the Pioneer Battalion. It is entitled 'Medical History of 2/1st Aust Pioneer Battalion. Medical Chapter.' Held by Sue Hallenstein.

52 As described by Chester Wilmot, when the moon was out, German bombers were able to see the silvery wake of the Allied ships as they approached the Tobruk harbour.

53 The Pioneer Battalion history records the deep appreciation that the Australian infantry had of the two navies and the British artillery force which helped to defend Tobruk.

54 Interview with Sue Hallenstein and Goulston's albums of photographs from the Middle East.

55 Copy of the Ballet and Music Concert programme held by Diana Goulston Robinson.

56 Osborn, *The Pioneers*, p. 184.

57 Ibid., p. 75.

58 As an officer, Goulston was possibly not limited to a telegram and could tell Jean where he was.

59 Robert Likeman, *The Thousand Doors: The Australian Doctors at War Series: Vol. Four: The Middle East and Far East 1929–42*, 2014.

60 The Australian Hospital Ship (AHS) *Centaur* was sunk by a Japanese submarine off the coast of Queensland in May 1943. Of the Army medical personnel and civilian crew on board, 268 out of 332 died. The deaths included 63 of the 65 Army staff, of whom several were doctors.

61 Video made by Jim Gerrand in 1999: *Dr Eric Goulston, 'Wrong Side of Seventy'*, which includes interviews with the three Goulston brothers – Eric, Stan and Roy.

62 In Greece, Eric Goulston was with the 2nd/5th Australian General Hospital, and – like Dr William Morrow, who took charge of the AGH when their superior officer was killed – was in great danger during the forced evacuation of the field hospital.

63 Goulston, 'A Doctor at War'.

64 This is a central stanza of a seven-verse poem entitled the 'Ode of Remembrance' and will be familiar to anyone who has attended an Anzac dawn service. The full poem may be found at https://en.wikisource.org/wiki/The_Times/1914/Arts/For_the_Fallen.

65 P. Braithwaite, 'The Regimental Medical Officer', *Medical Journal of Australia*, 1943, vol. 1, pp. 137–142. Braithwaite was an experienced Regimental Medical Officer, having served with the 2nd/12th Battalion throughout the siege of Tobruk. Likeman, *The Thousand Doors*, p. 38

5: Army Life after Tobruk

1 Material prepared by Goulston as his contribution to the written history of the Pioneer Battalion. It is entitled 'Medical History of 2/1st Aust Pioneer Battalion. Medical Chapter'. Held by Sue Hallenstein.

2 The Japanese Army began its attempt to occupy Port Moresby when forces were landed on the north coast of New Guinea on 21 July 1942, leading to the famous battles on the Kokoda Track.

3 Stan Goulston, interview, 2008.

4 Goulston later described this 'as the best exercise in training education that I've seen anywhere in my life in those Army days'.

5 Stan and Jean Goulston, interview. 2004. The husband of this couple was also serving in the Army.

6 Ibid.

7 Ibid.

8 S. Goulston, 'Talk Given to the NSW Jewish Ex-Servicemen and Women on Armistice Day, 1985'. Copy held by Diana Goulston Robinson.

9 K.J. Goulston, 'A Doctor, a Poet, and Many Other Roles [Obituary]', *Sydney Morning Herald*, 7 October 2011 and letter of reference to the Royal Prince Alfred Hospital from Colonel John H. Anderson, 1946.

10 S.J.M. Goulston, 'The Need for a Medical Liaison Officer in Peace and War', *Medical Journal of Australia*, 1947, vol. 2, pp. 329–332.

11 RMS *Queen Elizabeth* was built in 1938 as a luxury liner but was converted to a troop carrier for World War II. See https://en.wikipedia.org/wiki/RMS_Queen_Elizabeth#Second_World_War.

12 Goulston's reference to a 'second front' presumably refers to the D-Day, 6 June 1944 landing in Normandy of Allied Forces that led to the liberation of France.

13 John Buckley, *Recollections of the Roving Staff Officer*, 1993, p. 318.

14 Goulston wrote in 1947: '[I]n a global war it is essential that each member of an allied fighting team knows what the others are doing. The medical services are no exception.'

15 Goulston, 'The Need for a Medical Liaison Officer in Peace and War'.

16 Ibid.

17 Mass production methods in the USA made penicillin widely available to the military just ahead of the 1944 invasion of Normandy.

18 Stan Goulston, interview, 2008.

19 There were parallel offices for the Navy and Air Force Medical Services.

20 Goulston, 'The Need for a Medical Liaison Officer in Peace and War'.

21 Goulston, 'Talk Given to the NSW Jewish Ex-Servicemen and Women on Armistice Day, 1985'.

22 Ibid.

23 The case presented by his superiors for this award is detailed in Chapter 4 of this volume. The briefer citation at the award ceremony read 'Splendid example of courage and devotion in the Libya area'. Document held by Diana Goulston Robinson.

24 S.J.M. Goulston, 'The Malaria Frontline. Pioneering Malaria Research by the Australian Army in World War II [Letter]', *Medical Journal of Australia*, 1997, vol. 166, p. 672. Brigadier Hamilton Fairley's leadership of this vital research was recognised in Britain as, soon after the war ended, he was appointed Professor of Tropical Medicine at the London School of Hygiene and Tropical Medicine. Robert Likeman, *The Thousand Doors: The Australian Doctors at War Series: Vol. Four: The Middle East and Far East 1929–42*, 2014, p. 35.

25 Before the war, Colonel John H. Anderson, CMG, CBE, MD (Melb.) worked as Acting Professor of Anatomy at the University of Melbourne and held an Honorary Outpatient Physician appointment at St Vincent's Hospital, Melbourne. In 1946, he was working in Wales.

26 In 1946, Professor (later Sir) John McMichael, MD, FRCP was the Acting Director of the British Postgraduate Medical School at Hammersmith Hospital. Shortly afterwards he was confirmed as Director and served in that role for twenty years.

27 Brigadier Neil Hamilton Fairley, MD, FRCO, FRS, a graduate of the University of Melbourne, was appointed Professor of Tropical Medicine at the University of London soon after the war.

28 Jean Goulston, interview, 2004.

29 Goulston, 'The Need for a Medical Liaison Officer in Peace and War'.

30 Dr McMichael was appointed a Professor and Director of the Postgraduate Medical School in 1946.

31 Letter of recommendation written by Professor John McMichael in August 1946.

32 Stan Goulston, interview, 2008.

33 The first such liver biopsy was done in Australia in 1947 by Dr Bill King, working with Dr Ian Wood in Melbourne. V.D. Plueckhahn, 'Not an Armchair Pathologist – Inaugural John Perry Memorial Oration', *Pathology*, 1977, vol. 9, pp. 1–11.

34 Stan Goulston, interview, 2008.

35 Letter of recommendation written by Dr Sheila Sherlock in August 1946.

36 See https://en.wikipedia.org/wiki/RMS_Orion.

37 See https://www.holocaust.com.au/australia-and-the-european-theatres-of-war/.

6: Returning to Family Life

1 Jean recalls wearing her best clothes as well as a hat, gloves and bag when going to the synagogue.

2 Jean Goulston, interview, 2004.

3 As Jean remarked in 2004: 'But that's what fathers did in those days, they didn't take any part in any domesticity at all – no father ever did, no man did'.

4 Jean described her mother, May, as 'very capable – Dad relied on her for everything'.

5 Few homes had refrigerators so preservation of some foods depended on other methods. Ice for ice-chests was delivered three times a week, but ice-chests were not particularly effective.

6 Her mother taught Jean to knit from an early age. Jean hated sewing.

7 J.S. Levi, *Rabbi Jacob Danglow: The Uncrowned Monarch of Australian Jews*, 1995, p. 79.

8 Jean Goulston, interview, 2004.

9 Ibid.

10 Claire refused to attend Hebrew lessons and her parents did not force the issue.

11 Jean commented that Claire 'was a real character, she knew what she wanted and she got it'.

12 Stan recalled that these three months were 'very difficult times' but he did not enlarge further.

13 Diana Goulston Robinson, e-mail, 20 May 2020.

14 The loans were soon repaid.

15 Stan and Jean Goulston, interview 2004.

16 Sadhana Goulston, interview, 1 May 2020; Sue Hallenstein, e-mail, 19 May 2020.

17 Daughter Wendy recalled, 'Dad always taught us to rejoice in nature. He would take me round the garden before he went to work, pointing out little changes from yesterday.' Interview, 2008.

18 In a letter to daughter Diana dated 16 October 1977, Stan wrote: 'Our roses have exceeded anything we have ever had before in the first blooming flush – really magnificent prize winning roses full of tremendous vigour. Even Mike Gilmour, noted NZ rose grower, was really impressed – all due to mulch and cow manure!!'

19 Sadhana Goulston, interview, 1 May 2020 and Wendy Goulston, interview, 8 May 2020. Stan was generous with his flowers and they went as equally to important visitors as they did to his house-cleaners.

20 Stan Goulston, letter to daughter Diana, 16 October 1977.

21 Late in life, Stan remarked, 'Yes, Friday night was the closest one that came to being religious, I think'.

22 The North Sydney Demonstration School is a government primary with

academic links to the Education Faculty of the University of Sydney. See https://nthsyddem-p.schools.nsw.gov.au/about-our-school.html.

23 When the Goulston girls attended the school it was known as Presbyterian Ladies' College Pymble, founded in 1916 as a branch of Presbyterian Ladies' College Croydon. It is now Pymble Ladies' College, a private school of the Uniting Church in Australia. See https://www.pymblelc.nsw.edu.au/.

24 Wendy Goulston, interview, May 2020.

25 Daughter Sue remarked that her father 'was very good helping us with our homework when we were later in senior school – in maths and science'.

26 Sue also recalled a weekend when she was seeking help with French homework but her father gave her the choice of seeing a movie and they went off to *The Guns of Navarone*.

27 Stan Goulston recalled that 'we had a lot of music in the house'.

28 A daughter's e-mail, 28 April 2020.

29 Brother Eric was a keen golfer but Stan only played occasionally.

30 'Higgs, Jean Millicent (1912–2006)', https://trove.nla.gov.au/list?id=124294.

31 In an account that demonstrates Jean's generosity and thoughtfulness, medical friends, John and Alex Chalmers, described their experience when calling into visit when driving home from Queensland to South Australia with their five children aged eleven to six. Not only were they asked to stay the night, but they were welcomed with a fine roast dinner. Beside each child's plate was an individual pottery mug that Jean had made for them specially.

32 Zara Selby, interview, March 2020.

33 Lysbeth Cohen, *Beginning with Esther: Jewish Women in New South Wales from 1788*, 1987, pp. 426–428.

34 Stan described his wife as 'self-reliant, very calm, very rarely lost her temper'.

35 Dr Alex Bune, wife of John Chalmers, got to know Jean well and was much taken by the warmth apparent in Jean's eyes.

36 Wendy Goulston, interview, May 2020.

37 The ceremony for the girls was a form of group 'confirmation' rather than the modern, more elaborate ceremony.

38 That daughter chose to not have a Bat Mitzvah because the idea 'scared the daylights out of her'.

39 Brenda Niall, *Judy Cassab: A Portrait*, 2005.

40 Judy Cassab, *Judy Cassab Diaries*, 1995, p. 53.

41 Daughter Sue commented that 'Mum and Dad just had such an extraordinary relationship … the amount of pleasure and joy they got from each other is extraordinary'.

42 Daughter Diana felt that it was her mother's 'enormous patience, love, calmness and give and take' that made the marriage work. She also felt that her mother 'was unique' and that such a relationship would not be possible now.

43 Comment of daughter Sue, in 2008.

44 Stan may have understated the intensity of some of their arguments as their daughters recall times when their parents retired to their bedroom 'to have it out in private and reappear both looking pretty grim'.

45 Stan had long thought about the point in time when the girls would leave home and had resolved that 'provided it was for their own good and their life, one should be joyous about it rather than worry about them not being around'. Interview, 2004.

46 Her daughters recalled that Jean's parents would not allow Jean to travel alone and she adored travel, and that from a young age, Jean had taught them 'what a great thing travel was'.

47 Stan Goulston, interview, 2008.

7: Honorary Physician to the Royal Prince Alfred Hospital

1 *Royal Prince Alfred Hospital: 125 Year Anniversary Book*, 2007, pp. 127–148; M.K. Doherty, edited by R.L. Russell, *The Life and Times of Royal Prince Alfred Hospital, Sydney*, 1996.

2 As discussed in Chapter 8, in 1962 the strict insistence on referral to a matching surgical unit was overturned for patients with severe ulcerative colitis and this led to striking improvement in outcomes. *Royal Prince Alfred Hospital: 125 Year Anniversary Book*. p. 136.

3 The notion of not making permanent appointments had been advised by a joint wartime committee of the Royal Australasian College of Surgeons and the Royal Australasian College of Physicians. R. Winton. *Why the Pomegranate? A History of the Royal College of Physicians of Australasia*, 1988, p. 32.

4 The four Sydney teaching hospitals (RPAH, Sydney Hospital, St Vincent's Hospital and Royal North Shore Hospital) made no senior appointments during the war. By this policy, the hospitals encouraged their senior staff to enlist and reassured them that they would not be disadvantaged on their return.

5 Col. John H. Anderson, CMG, CBE, MD (Melb.), JP, then working in Wales but previously Acting Professor of Anatomy at the University of Melbourne and Honorary Outpatient Physician at St Vincent's Hospital, Melbourne.

6 Dr J. McMichael, MD, FRCP, Acting Director British Postgraduate Medical School, Hammersmith Hospital. Letter dated 2 September 1946.

7 Dr N. Hamilton Fairley, MD, FRCO, FRS, Professor of Tropical Medicine, University of London. Letter dated 19 August 1946.

8 Dr Sheila Sherlock, MD, MRCP, Assistant Physician, British Postgraduate Medical School, Hammersmith Hospital. Letter dated August 1946.

9 Dr John Halliday, MRCP, FRACP, Assistant Physician, RPAH. Letter dated 11 September 1946.

10 Dr W.P. MacCallum, MB ChM, MRACP, Honorary at Royal Alexandra Hospital for Children, Honorary at RPAH, Late Brigadier, Deputy Director General of Medical Services, HQ, Australian Military Forces. Letter dated 24 August 1946.

11 Dr A.W. Morrow, Formerly Consultant Physician, Advanced Headquarters, Australian Military Forces. Letter dated 18 August 1946.

12 Dr Kempson Maddox, MD, MRCP, FRACP. Letter dated 18 April 1946.

13 Dr Lorimer Dodds, MD, DCH, FRACP. Letter dated 16 September 1946. Dodds had worked with Goulston abroad as well as in Darwin and at Concord Hospital, Sydney.

14 Dr Charles Kellaway, MBBS, MD, MS, had served as Director of the Walter and Eliza Hall Institute in Melbourne but in 1944 took up the post of Director of Scientific Policy for the Wellcome Foundation in London, where he met Dr Goulston. Letter dated 20 August 1946.

15 As no appointments had been made during the war, four vacancies were advertised. These physicians were to replace older doctors who had come out of retirement to help the hospital during the war.

16 Goulston estimated that close to 50% of his working week was honorary, as was that of the other physicians at RPAH who were helping to develop the specialties of cardiology, respiratory medicine and renal medicine. Interview, 2008.

17 Goulston appreciated the status of being on RPAH staff in terms of 'you were made', as the hospital was 'the leader then in everything'. Interview, 2008.

18 For popular and highly regarded specialists, doctors and their families could constitute a significant proportion of patients. In lieu of paying an account, doctors and their families who received this courtesy felt duty bound to give the doctor a gift. One prominent Sydney obstetrician made sure that his secretary instructed such patients that he would like to receive Waterford crystal.

19 Daughter Sue recalls going to the airport when Goulston flew to see patients in the country. Goulston noted that this was 'quite common in those days' and recalled Sir William Morrow and Sir Thomas Greenaway going on the weekends to places like Taree or Mudgee, to see two or three patients for generous fees. Interview, 2008.

20 J. Hassall, *RPA & Beyond: An Unauthorised Memoir*, 2010.

21 Ruth Teale, 'Schlink, Sir Herbert Henry (1883–1962)', *Australian Dictionary of Biography*, http://adb.anu.edu.au/biography/schlink-sir-herbert-henry-8359/text14551, published first in hardcopy 1988.

22 'Dr Thomas Greenaway, 1902–1980', https://www.racp.edu.au/about/college-roll/college-roll-bio/greenaway-i-sir-i-thomas-moore.

23 'Dr William "Billy" Bye, 1901–1967', https://www.racp.edu.au/about/college-roll/college-roll-bio/bye-william-alick. Dr Bye was a prisoner of war at Changi and received an OBE for his work supporting fellow prisoners.

24 Dr Warwick Selby, interview, April 2020.

25 Professor John Chalmers described Goulston as 'one of the humblest and gentlest people' and added that he was 'one of the great figures in Medicine and one of the finest men I have known'. E-mail, 23 January 2020.

26 Dr Selby, if irked by a situation or a patient and inclined to show it, would silently remind himself that 'Stan would not do that, why would I do it?' Interview, April 2020.

27 Emeritus Professor John Chalmers, interview, April 2020.

28 Dr Miles Little, interview, 29 April 2020.

29 A medical student from the 1950s, Ben Nebenzahl, in a letter to Sadhana Goulston in September 2020, remembered him as a 'kind, knowledgeable, sensitive' teacher who was 'an inspiration to us all'.

30 Dr J. Schneeweiss – AM, FRACP, a consultant physician in Sydney – letter to the Goulston family, 2 November 2011. Dr Schneeweiss died in 2017.

31 When a colleague of Goulston's, Professor Miles Little, stepped down from the Chair of Surgery at Westmead Hospital with the plan of establishing a medical ethics centre at the University of Sydney, Goulston lent strong support while other colleagues were sceptical. Emeritus Professor Miles Little, interview, 29 April 2020.

32 Kerry Goulston, interview March 2020.

33 John Chalmers, interview April 2020.

34 Goulston conducted these teaching rounds from 1961 until 1970 when he was made Censor-in-Chief.

35 Dr Michael Pain, e-mail 11 March 2020. Dr Pain was also impressed by Goulston's 'evident enjoyment in his profession', such that it helped to confirm Pain's decision to become a physician.

36 Professor Miles Little, interview, 29 April 2020. As a student, Little had presented a well-worked-up case to Blackburn and received the brunt of what was probably a misconceived approach to teaching by Blackburn. Later in the teaching round, Goulston drew Little aside and told him, 'Don't listen to him, you did well'.

37 K.J. Breen, S.M. Cordner and C.H. Thomson, *Good Medical Practice: Professionalism, Ethics and Law*, 4th edn, 2016, p. 21.

38 Stan Goulston, letter to daughter Diana, 28 April 1977.

39 Goulston did benefit from a rule change in 1974 when the retirement age of honorary medical staff was raised from sixty to sixty-five years.

40 Goulston shared a weekly gastroscopy list with Dr Warwick Selby for some years. Warwick Selby, interview, April 2020.

41 Hassall, *RPA & Beyond*, p. 27.

42 At St Vincent's Hospital, Melbourne and at the Royal Melbourne Hospital, despite the demands for specialist beds, a strong general medical presence has been maintained. Many teaching hospitals have regretted the decision to abandon general medical units.

8: Gastroenterology and the Gastroenterological Society of Australia

1 As time passed, the general medical component of his private practice diminished and the gastroenterology component grew such that in the last few years, after he had retired from RPAH, he was practising as a gastroenterologist. Dr Kerry Goulston, interview, 25 March 2020.

2 In addition to Goulston, other physicians in charge of general units at RPAH in the 1960s included Richard Harris and John Sands.

3 Graham Macdonald, 'Sands, John Robert (1919–1980)', *Australian Dictionary of*

Biography, http://adb.anu.edu.au/biography/sands-john-robert-11612/text20735, published first in hardcopy 2002.

4 See https://www.mapmycareer.health.nsw.gov.au/Pages/specialty-details.aspx?specialty=50§ion=ms.

5 Although Goulston acknowledged the major contributions of Ian Wood to the development of gastroenterology in Australia in his 1970 review, the Clinical Research Unit at the Royal Melbourne Hospital never claimed to be a specialised gastroenterology unit. After Ian Wood retired, this was even more apparent as the interests of the unit narrowed to immune diseases, including Ian Mackay's 'lupoid hepatitis'.

6 S. Goulston and M. Smith, 'Intrahepatic Biliary Obstruction of Unknown Origin', *Medical Journal of Australia*, 1951, vol. 2, pp. 313–317 and S. Goulston, 'Experience with Infectious Hepatitis at Royal Prince Alfred Hospital', *Medical Journal of Australia*, 1953, vol. 1, pp. 905–913.

7 Neil Gallagher, 'Morrow, Sir Arthur William (Bill) (1903–1977)', *Australian Dictionary of Biography*, http://adb.anu.edu.au/biography/morrow-sir-arthur-william-bill-11178/text19919, published first in hardcopy 2000.

8 Like Sydney Grammar School, Newington College is a member of the Sydney Greater Public Schools Association.

9 Readers not familiar with the traditional practice of Sydney University may be puzzled by Morrow's year of graduation being the same year as his junior medical residency. While his final year of the medical course was 1926, his official graduation took place early in 1927.

10 In that era, clinical superintendent and deputy clinical superintendent positions were akin to the modern registrar. Rather than being administrative positions, their role was to support and guide the resident doctors between the infrequent attendance of the honorary senior medical staff.

11 For the Allied Forces campaign in Greece in 1942, the 6th AIF Division, now battle hardened from its time in Libya, was sent to assist. Lacking adequate armaments and with little air support, the Allies were overrun by the Germans and forced to retreat in difficult circumstances.

12 The colleague was Dr Neil Gallagher, who served as Director of the Morrow Unit at RPAH from 1973 to 1998.

13 See http://sydney.edu.au/medicine/museum/mwmuseum/index.php/Morrow,_Sir_Arthur_William and Robert Likeman, *The Thousand Doors: The Australian Doctors at War Series: Vol. Four: The Middle East and Far East 1929–42*, 2014, p. 284.

14 N.D. Gallagher (ed.), *The A.W. Morrow Unit: 50 Years of Australian Gastroenterology at Royal Prince Alfred Hospital, 1948–1998*, 1998.

15 All medical inpatients in the wards of RPAH were under the care and control of the honorary physician to each of the medical units. No other senior clinician could approach an inpatient without the permission of the physician-in-charge. When invited to do so, the second physician was 'consulting' for the purpose of giving advice. Very occasionally the consulting specialist was then invited to take over the management of the case.

16 See https://www.165macquariestreet.com.au/. The Sydney-based Australian Club has reciprocal arrangements with the Melbourne Club.

17 Sir William Slim was Governor General of Australia between 1953 and 1959. He served in the British Army in both world wars and rose to Field Marshall. As he had served alongside Australian troops at Gallipoli, he was a popular choice as Governor General. His Army service may well have been a reason for his bond with Morrow. See https://en.wikipedia.org/wiki/William_Slim,_1st_Viscount_Slim.

18 'A Tribute to Sir William Morrow', in Gallagher (ed.), *The A.W. Morrow Unit*, p. 3.

19 The friendship apparently developed after Morrow had successfully treated Bushell for a serious illness. Gallagher (ed.). *The A.W. Morrow Unit*, p. 2.

20 Philip Bushell was a successful Australian tea merchant and philanthropist. In the 1940s, he and his family founded the Bushell Trust which donated funds to medical research and medical education. Bill Morrow was one of the trustees. G.P. Walsh, 'Bushell, Philip Howard (1879–1954)', *Australian Dictionary of Biography*, http://adb.anu.edu.au/biography/bushell-philip-howard-5439/text9233, published first in hardcopy 1979.

21 Former physician trainee at RPAH, Dr Alex Bune, praised Morrow's care of her dying grand-aunt and recalled that her mother, also a doctor, had only good words to say about Morrow as a physician. Interview, April 2008.

22 Dr Allan Cooke, interview, April 2020.

23 The respect and affection that Goulston held for Morrow is evident in the entry that Goulston wrote for the RACP College Roll after Morrow's death in 1997. See https://www.racp.edu.au/about/college-roll/college-roll-bio/sir-arthur-william-morrow.

24 Former trainees Allan Cooke and Kerry Goulston both held this view.

25 The differences in temperament between the Morrow and Goulston led one former trainee to write, 'In a sense they were an odd couple but worked well together'.

26 Late in life, Goulston was asked if Morrow had ever nominated him for membership of the Australian Club. His reply was 'no, but I didn't mind that really … I didn't want to belong to that club. I belonged to the University Club which was a good club anyway.' Interview, 2008.

27 Dr Jim Rankin's description of this large table suggests that it was the type used in a linen room or sewing room, so perhaps it had been used for that purpose.

28 Dr Jim Rankin, interview, April 2020.

29 The Herman Taylor gastroscope was an improvement on the earlier Schindler instrument in that the flexible lower end was directable, thereby reducing the number of blind spots. W. Sircus, 'Milestones in the Evolution of Endoscopy: A Short History', *Journal of the Royal College of Physicians of Edinburgh*, 2003, vol. 33, pp. 124–134.

30 This semi-rigid gastroscope, a major advance in its time, was the creation of Dr Rudolf Schindler and German instrument-maker Georg Wolf and was first demonstrated in Munich in 1932. It was first used in Australia in 1937 by Dr

John Horan at St Vincent's Hospital in Melbourne, who later taught Sir Ian Wood how to use it. J. Horan, 'Gastroscopy', *Medical Journal of Australia*, 1937, vol. 2, pp. 243–248.

31 Individuals are appointed a Companion of the Order of Australia (AC) for eminent achievement and merit of the highest degree in service to Australia or to humanity at large. See https://www.gg.gov.au/australian-honours-and-awards/order-australia.

32 'Professor Charles Ruthven Bickerton Blackburn (1913–2016)', http://sydney.edu.au/medicine/museum/mwmuseum/index.php/Blackburn,_Charles_Ruthven_Bickerton.

33 Dr Brian Morgan, interview, May 2020.

34 Morrow had to give up his honorary appointment when he reached the age of sixty. However, he was made welcome in the GE Unit for many more years and would perform one or two gastroscopies on his private patients early on a Monday morning, assisted by the unit registrar.

35 Dr McCredie had performed a barium enema X-ray on a Dutchman who had lived in Indonesia and had been imprisoned by the Japanese during World War II. The patient suffered long-standing bowel symptoms and was referred to Goulston. McCredie found a 'conical caecum' and quickly ascertained that this was typical scarring of long-standing amoebic colitis, an infection rarely seen in Australia. She called Goulston, who attended promptly, examined the X-rays with her and then went to see his pathology colleague, Dr McGovern, to have the patient's rectal biopsy reviewed. There under the microscope were the amoebae, missed on the first examination. Dr Janet McCredie, interview, 20 May 2020.

36 US manufacturer ACMI began manufacturing fibre-optic endoscopes ahead of the Japanese but eventually failed to match the quality of Olympus gastroscopes and colonoscopes.

37 Morgan clearly recalled their discussions. Having been given the wonderful news that he and the colonoscope were to be made welcome in the GE Unit, he then thought to ask 'but what about paying for it?' The reply came from Sir William, 'leave that to me'. Dr Brian Morgan, interview, 20 May 2020.

38 Before the advent of the fibre-optic gastroscope, it was not possible to biopsy lesions in the stomach using the semi-rigid gastroscope. To seek evidence of gastric cancer, a soft nasogastric tube was passed and the stomach was lavaged with a large quantity of fluid. The recovered fluid was centrifuged and the cellular deposit examined microscopically – a task requiring patience, thoroughness and experience.

39 Dr Brian Morgan, interview, 20 May 2020.

40 This is a topic worthy of more research but the general physicians in every Australian teaching hospital in this era felt threatened by the emergence of specialists and found ways to delay or obstruct their deployment.

41 'Brian Brooke. Obituary', https://www.independent.co.uk/arts-entertainment/obituary-professor-bryan-brooke-1175817.html.

42 'Burrill Crohn, Obituary', https://www.nytimes.com/1983/07/30/obituaries/dr-burrill-b-crohn-99-an-expert-on-diseases-of-the-intestinal-tract.html.

43 'Portrait Marks Gastro Transition', *Pacemaker* (Staff News Sheet of the RPAH), 1983, November, vol. 14, no. 2, p. 2.

44 Stan Goulston, letter to daughter Diana, 6 July 1991.

45 Diana Robinson (née Goulston), e-mail 28 April 2020.

46 The British Society of Gastroenterology was founded by Dr Hurst in 1937 as the Gastroenterological Club and had a restricted membership of forty physicians plus one pathologist, one biochemist, one radiologist and one surgeon. In 1945, the group renamed itself the British Society of Gastroenterologists and membership was enlarged. In 1949, the name was changed again to the British Society of Gastroenterology. See https://www.bsg.org.uk/about/history-of-the-bsg/.

47 See https://www.gastro.org/about-aga/about-us.

48 J.C. Wiseman (ed.), *To Follow Knowledge: A History of Examinations, Continuing Education and Specialist Affiliations of the Royal Australasian College of Physicians*, 1988.

49 E. Russell and K. Sheedy, *A Passion for the Gut: The Evolution of Gastroenterology in Australia*, 2009, p. 9.

50 For example, the Haematology Society of Australia, formed in 1961, arose from a Melbourne group, the Blood Club. K.J. Breen, *The Man We Never Knew: Carl de Gruchy – Medical Pioneer*, 2019, p. 99.

51 Interview of Dr Stan Goulston, conducted by Dr Greg Whelan in 1990 for the archives of the Gastroenterological Society of Australia. Summary kindly provided by historian Emma Russell.

52 Information provided by Karen Myers, Librarian at the RACP.

53 The choice of the title 'Society' and not 'Association' probably reflects the strong links that Australian physicians then had with Britain.

54 Goulston explained that Sir Ian Wood 'was felt to be the father figure and leader in the field. He was approached ... but he constantly declined the honour'. Russell and Sheedy, *A Passion for the Gut*, p. 12.

55 Ibid.

56 Minutes of the Adelaide meeting. Copy published in Gallagher (ed.), *The A.W. Morrow Unit*, at p. 47.

57 Russell and Sheedy, *A Passion for the Gut*, p. 9.

58 Ibid., p. 44. The World Gastroenterology Organisation was originally called the Organisation Mondiale de Gastro-entérologie. The name change took place in 2007.

59 ERCP stands for endoscopic retrograde cholangiopancreatography. By this remarkable advance, excellent images of the bile duct, gallbladder and pancreas were obtained via gastro-duodenoscopy and soon instruments were designed to allow gallstones to be removed without major abdominal surgery.

9: Clinical Researcher and Academic

1 Until the 1970s, nearly all senior medical and surgical appointments to Royal Prince Alfred Hospital (RPAH) and similar teaching hospitals across Australia were

honorary and part-time. Even after sessional payment was introduced, it remained rare for visiting medical officers such as Goulston to be involved in research and publication of findings. Research was never part of the job description or the expectation of the Health Department which funded their positions.

2 S.J.M. Goulston, 'A Regimental Aid Post in Tobruk', *Medical Journal of Australia*, 1942, vol. 1, pp. 494–496.

3 See, for example, 'Chemical Warfare: Compiled under the Direction of the Committee on the Survey of War Medicine of the National Health and Medical Research Council', *Medical Journal of Australia*, 1943, vol. 1, pp. 29–32.

4 E. Goulston, 'Guerrilla Surgery', *Medical Journal of Australia*, 1942, vol. 2, pp. 134–136.

5 P. Braithwaite, 'The Regimental Medical Officer', *Medical Journal of Australia*, 1943, vol. 1, pp. 137–142.

6 T.L. Tyers, 'A New Method of Radiological Localization of Foreign Bodies', *Medical Journal of Australia*, 1942, vol. 1, pp. 493–494.

7 F.R. Hone, E.V. Keogh and R. Andrew, 'Bacillary Dysentery in an Australian Hospital in the Middle East'. *Medical Journal of Australia*, 1942, vol. 1, pp. 631–635.

8 E.L. Cooper, 'Relapsing Fever in Tobruk', *Medical Journal of Australia*, 1942, vol. 1, pp. 635–637. The first author, Lieutenant Colonel Eric Cooper, served with the 2/4th Army Hospital in Tobruk and returned to Australia in February 1942. He died in May 1942 of septicaemia before his paper was published. Robert Likeman, *The Thousand Doors: The Australian Doctors at War Series: Vol. Four: The Middle East and Far East 1929–42*, 2014, p. 16.

9 E.L. Cooper and A.J.M. Sinclair, 'War Neuroses in Tobruk: A Report on 207 Patients from the Australian Imperial Force Units in Tobruk', *Medical Journal of Australia*, 1942, vol. 2, pp. 73–77.

10 H.R. Love, 'Dyspeptic Symptoms in Soldiers', *Medical Journal of Australia*, 1943, vol. 2, pp. 101–109.

11 J.F. McCulloch, 'Anaesthesia under Wartime Conditions', *Medical Journal of Australia*, 1943, vol. 2, pp. 81–83, and S.V. Marshall, 'Further Aspects of Anaesthesia under Wartime Conditions', *Medical Journal of Australia*, 1943, vol. 2, pp. 83–85.

12 J. Devine, 'A Note on Desert Sores', *Medical Journal of Australia*, 1943, vol. 2, pp. 261–262.

13 'Clinical Meeting in the Middle East, *Medical Journal of Australia*, 1942, vol. 2, pp. 14–17, and 'Clinical Meeting at 2/11 Australian General Hospital', *Medical Journal of Australia*, 1942, vol. 2, pp. 470–473.

14 *Medical Journal of Australia*, 1947, vol. 2, pp. 329–332.

15 His paper helped to inform Chapter 5.

16 At that time, the British Medical Association was the equivalent of the Australian Medical Association (AMA). The AMA was officially formed in 1962.

17 S. Goulston, 'Recent Advances in Medicine in England', *Medical Journal of Australia*, 1947, vol. 2, pp. 8–10.

18 Writing only of 'medical men' was an unfortunate slip as Goulston was well aware that one of the emerging leaders in the field was Dr Sheila Sherlock.

19 The British Postgraduate School of Medicine, established in1935, was later renamed the Royal Postgraduate Medical School. It was based at the Hammersmith Hospital and its academic staff were also the senior consultants to the hospital.

20 Dr (later Sir) Francis Avery-Jones was based at the Central Middlesex Hospital and in the 1940s and 1950s was one of the best known specialists in gastroenterology in the UK. He wrote a popular textbook on the subject. See https://www.independent.co.uk/news/obituaries/obituary-sir-francis-avery-jones-1159805.html.

21 Professor (later Sir) George Pickering was Head of St Mary's Hospital Medical School in London and later was Regius Professor of Medicine at the University of Oxford from 1956 to 1968. He was particularly known for his research into hypertension and was one of the most respected medical academics of his era. See http://munksroll.rcplondon.ac.uk/Biography/Details/3556.

22 Professor (later Sir) John McMichael served as Director of the Postgraduate School of Medicine from 1946 to 1966. His specialty was cardiology. See https://en.wikipedia.org/wiki/Sir_John_McMichael.

23 Dr Sheila Sherlock, as she was known to Goulston, became a Professor of Medicine at the Royal Free Hospital. She wrote a well-known textbook on liver diseases, first published in 1955, and went on to be internationally known and respected for her expertise. Many Australian doctors trained under her over the years. See https://en.wikipedia.org/wiki/Sheila_Sherlock.

24 S. Goulston and M. Smith, 'Intrahepatic Biliary Obstruction of Unknown Origin', *Medical Journal of Australia*, 1951, vol. 2, pp. 313–317.

25 The GE Unit later reported in detail many instances of what they called 'pericholangitis', now better known as intrahepatic sclerosing cholangitis.

26 S. Goulston, 'Experience with Infectious Hepatitis at Royal Prince Alfred Hospital', *Medical Journal of Australia*, 1953, vol. 1, pp. 905–913.

27 S. Goulston, 'The Treatment of Peptic Ulceration', *Medical Journal of Australia*, 1952, vol. 1, pp. 291–293. Also S. Goulston and M. Smith, 'An Analysis of the Value of Medical Care in a Group of Repatriation Male Duodenal Ulcer Patients', *Australasian Annals of Medicine*, 1955, vol. 4, pp. 255–260, and P.J. Crowe and S. Goulston, 'Post-gastrectomy Dietary Management', *Medical Journal of Australia*, 1954, vol. 2, pp. 430–433.

28 S. Goulston, 'Management of Hiatus Hernia', *Australian and New Zealand Journal of Surgery*, 1956, vol. 26, pp. 101–105.

29 S. Goulston, 'The Value and Limitations of X-ray Examination in Assessing Disease of the Gall-bladder', *Medical Journal of Australia*, 1952, vol. 1, pp. 323–325.

30 S.P. Mistilis and C.R. Blackburn, 'The Treatment of Active Chronic Hepatitis with 6-Mercaptopurine and Azathioprine', *Australasian Annals of Medicine*, 1967 November, vol. 16, no. 4, pp. 305–311; S.P. Mistilis, A.P. Skyring and C.R. Blackburn, 'Natural History of Active Chronic Hepatitis. I. Clinical Features,

Course, Diagnostic Criteria, Morbidity, Mortality and Survival', *Australasian Annals of Medicine*, 1968 August, vol. 17, no. 3, pp. 214–223; S.P. Mistilis, 'Natural History of Active Chronic Hepatitis. II. Pathology, Pathogenesis and Clinico-pathological Correlation', *Australasian Annals of Medicine*, 1968 November, vol. 17, no. 4, pp. 277–288; S.P. Mistilis and C.R. Blackburn, 'Active Chronic Hepatitis', *American Journal of Medicine*, 1970 April, vol. 48, no. 4, pp. 484–495.

31 At RPAH, there was close cooperation between the GE Unit and the Clinical Research Unit that Blackburn had developed. In 1957, Blackburn was appointed Professor of Medicine at the University of Sydney and provided distinguished service for many years. In his new role, he maintained a deep interest in this form of chronic liver disease. See https://www.sydney.edu.au/medicine/museum/mwmuseum/index.php/Blackburn,_Charles_Ruthven_Bickerton.

32 Goulston remained aware of this valuable wartime research and in 1997 reminded the medical profession of it via a brief letter in the *Medical Journal of Australia* (vol. 166, p. 67), where he commended the work of Blackburn and pointed out that the research findings had also been of value in the British fighting against the Japanese in Burma.

33 The other two lecturers were Dr Doug Piper, based at Royal North Shore Hospital and Dr John Hickie, at St Vincent's Hospital. See https://www.sydney.edu.au/medicine/museum/mwmuseum/index.php/Blackburn,_Charles_Ruthven_Bickerton.

34 Dr Vincent McGovern (1915–1983) was a graduate of the University of Otago in New Zealand and came to Australia in 1940, where he worked as a Resident Medical Officer for a year. He then joined the Australian Imperial Force and the Army sent him for training in pathology. After the war, he was appointed a pathologist at RPAH in 1950 and in 1959 was made director of the department. In 1977, the University of Sydney appointed him to a personal chair. Among many honours, he was elected President of the College of Pathologists of Australasia in 1975. In addition to his work with Goulston, he was also internationally recognised for his work in melanoma. He died prematurely in a car accident. A. Johnson, 'Obituary. Vincent John McGovern', *Australasian Journal of Dermatology*, 1984, vol. 25, pp. 35–36.

35 S.J. Goulston, 'A Personal Appreciation of Dr Vincent McGovern', *Pathology*, 1985, vol. 2, p. 151.

36 Ibid.

37 V.J. McGovern and S.J. Goulston, 'Crohn's Disease of the Colon', *Gut*, 1968, vol. 2, pp. 164–176.

38 S. Goulston, 'Ischaemic Colitis', *Medical Journal of Australia*, 1973, vol. 1, pp. 1194–1197.

39 S.J. Goulston and V.J. McGovern, 'Clinical Settings in Pseudomembranous Colitis', *Australian and New Zealand Journal of Medicine*, 1980, vol. 10, pp. 139–145.

40 Goulston, 'A Personal Appreciation of Dr Vincent McGovern', p. 151. Also S.J.M. Goulston and V.J. McGovern, 'Pseudo-membranous Colitis', *Gut*, 1965, vol. 6, pp. 207–212.

41 S.J. Goulston and V.J. McGovern, 'The Nature of Benign Strictures in Ulcerative Colitis', *New England Journal of Medicine*, 1969, vol. 281, pp. 290–295.

42 B. Morson, 'Muscle Abnormality in Ulcerative Colitis', *New England Journal of Medicine*, 1969, vol. 281, pp. 325–326.

43 S.J.M. Goulston and V.J. McGovern, *Fundamentals of Colitis*, 1981.

44 Captain James Cook was awarded the Copley Medal for his success in controlling scurvy on his long voyages of discovery. The Copley Medal was first awarded in 1731 and is the most prestigious award made by the Royal Society. See https://royalsociety.org/grants-schemes-awards/awards/copley-medal/.

45 S. Goulston and K. Breen, 'Gastroenterology in Australia. 1949–1969', *Postgraduate Medical Journal*, 1970, vol. 46, pp. 210–220.

46 This title reflects the power that the general physicians held at that time and is discussed in Chapter 7.

47 J.G. Rankin, S.J.M. Goulston, R.W. Boden and A.W. Morrow, 'Fulminant Ulcerative Colitis', *Quarterly Journal of Medicine*, 1960, vol. 29, pp. 375–389. Also N.D. Gallagher, S.J.M. Goulston, N. Wyndham and Sir William Morrow, 'The Management of Fulminant Ulcerative Colitis', *Gut*, 1962, vol. 3, pp. 306–311.

48 C.R. Vickers, N.D. Gallagher, D.C. Glenn, P. Morgan and S.J. Goulston, 'A Reappraisal of the Management of Severe Colitis in Its Fulminant Phase', *Journal of Gastroenterology and Hepatology*, 1987, vol. 2, no. 3, pp. 217–223.

49 R.W. Boden, J.G. Rankin, S.J.M. Goulston and A.W. Morrow, 'The Liver in Ulcerative Colitis', *Lancet*, 1959, vol. ii, pp. 245–248. Also J.G. Rankin, R.W. Boden, S.J.M. Goulston and A.W. Morrow, 'The Liver in Ulcerative Colitis. Treatment of Pericholangitis with Tetracycline', *Lancet*, 1959, vol. ii, pp. 1110–1112.

50 S.P. Mistilis, 'Pericholangitis and Ulcerative Colitis. I. Pathology, Etiology and Pathogenesis', *Annals of Internal Medicine*, 1965, vol. 63, pp. 1–16; S.P. Mistilis, A.P. Skyring and S.J.M. Goulston, 'Pericholangitis and Ulcerative Colitis. II. Clinical Aspects', *Annals of Internal Medicine*, 1965, vol. 63, pp. 17–26; S.P. Mistilis and S.J.M. Goulston, 'Liver Disease in Ulcerative Colitis', in B.N. Brooke (ed.), *Recent Advances in Gastroenterology*, 1965.

51 K.N. Lazaridis and N.F. LaRusso, 'Primary Sclerosing Cholangitis', *New England Journal of Medicine*, 2016, vol. 375, pp. 1161–1170.

52 S.J. Goulston, 'The Influence of the Royal Australasian College of Physicians on Physician Training and Evaluation. 1', *Medical Journal of Australia*, 1974, vol. 1, pp. 203–209; S.J. Goulston, 'The Influence of the Royal Australasian College of Physicians on Physician Training and Evaluation. 2', *Medical Journal of Australia*, 1974, vol. 1, pp. 247–254; S. Goulston, 'Control of Drug Usage', *Medical Journal of Australia*, 1981, vol. 1, pp. 166–168.

53 Goulston and McGovern, 'Clinical Settings in Pseudomembranous Colitis'. Also N.D. Gallagher and S.J. Goulston, 'Antibiotic Associated Colitis: In Search of a Cause and Treatment', *Drugs*, 1978, vol. 16, pp. 385–386; E.R. Smith and S.J. Goulston, 'Antibiotic-induced Diarrhoea', *Drugs*, 1975, vol. 10, pp. 329–332; S.J. Goulston and V.J. McGovern, 'The Value of Rectal Biopsies', *Medical Journal of Australia*, 1972, vol. 1, pp. 1234–1238.

54 'Centenary Convocation', *RPA Magazine*, 1983, Spring edition, pp. 4–5.

55 'Degree of Doctor of Medicine (Honoris Causa)', RACP *Fellowship Affairs Newsletter*, November 1983, vol. 2, no. 4, p. 8.

10: The Royal Australasian College of Physicians

1 This summary is drawn from the 1998 history written to mark the first fifty years of the RACP. R. Winton, *Why the Pomegranate? A History of the Royal College of Physicians of Australasia*, 1988.

2 This pathway applied to most of the contemporaries of Morrow and Goulston, but the pair were the exceptions as neither ever worked in general practice.

3 The medical schools were in Melbourne, Sydney, Adelaide and Brisbane.

4 The terms 'censor' and 'board of censors' were copied from the Royal College of Physicians of London. The role was to act as an examiner for entry to the college. In the 1980s, this arcane terminology was dropped and the group became known as the Committee for Clinical Examinations.

5 The Board of Censors was a small group and was seen to represent the elite of the college. One past examination candidate spoke of its 'magisterial remoteness'. Emeritus Professor Stephen Leeder, interview, April 2020.

6 S.J.M. Goulston, 'The Influence of the Royal Australasian College of Physicians on Physician Training and Evaluation: Part 1', *Medical Journal of Australia*, 1974, vol. 1, pp. 203–209; and S.J.M. Goulston, 'The Influence of the Royal Australasian College of Physicians on Physician Training and Evaluation: Part 2', *Medical Journal of Australia*, 1974, vol. 1, pp. 247–254.

7 J.C. Wiseman (ed.), *To Follow Knowledge: A History of Examinations, Continuing Education and Specialist Affiliations of the Royal Australasian College of Physicians*, 1998.

8 A 'long case' refers to the expectation that a candidate will spend an hour with a patient never seen before to take a detailed history, complete a full physical examination and prepare his or her thoughts on diagnosis and management ahead of presenting the case to a pair of examiners.

9 A 'short case' refers to the expectation that a candidate will conduct a brief but thorough physical examination of a designated body system (e.g., the cardiovascular system) while being observed by a pair of examiners and then present the findings orally to the examiners.

10 For example, Goulston passed the MRACP examination in 1944 and was made a Fellow (FRACP) in 1960.

11 It was always misleading to talk about a 'pass mark' for the written examination. It was an examination meant to filter out those who were deemed not yet ready to sit the clinical component.

12 Goulston, 'The Influence of the Royal Australasian College of Physicians on Physician Training and Evaluation: Part 1'.

13 Information provided by Ms Karen Myers, Librarian at the RACP.

14 'Board of Censors', *Australian and New Zealand Journal of Medicine*, 1974, vol. 4, no. 2, p. 218.

15 This eventually became a stressful task for the examiners when a decision was made that, to be fairer to the candidates, the examiners were to examine each patient 'blind' – i.e., without being told what the diagnosis was or what the agreed physical findings were. Now they felt that they were being examined!

16 For Goulston, the link with Singapore had begun much earlier, as in 1963 he had participated in the first advanced medicine course held there. Document held by Dr Kerry Goulston.

17 See https://ahha.asn.au/about-sidney-sax.

18 Copy of Dr Goulston's address to the Royal College of Physicians and Surgeons of Canada, Winnipeg, 23 January 1975. As RACP Censor-in-Chief, Goulston had attended a workshop on the international sharing of examination material held at the Ciba Foundation in London in 1972. Copy of address held by Dr Kerry Goulston.

19 Copy of the citation for honorary fellowship held by Dr Kerry Goulston.

20 Maori culture has a ceremony where a host lays down a challenge stick in front of a visitor. The visitor is expected to pick up the challenge stick to show that he comes in friendship.

21 Summary of Professor Hudson's 1984 speech provided by Ms Karen Myers, Librarian at the RACP.

22 Brenda Niall, *Judy Cassab: A Portrait*, 2005.

23 M. Davey, 'College of Physicians under Investigation after Years of Reported Dysfunction', https://www.theguardian.com/australia-news/2019/may/03/college-of-physicians-under-investigation-after-years-of-reported-dysfunction.

11: Other Service to the Community and the Medical Profession

1 The Sydney Grammar School magazine, *The Sydneian*, noted that he joined Legacy in 1949.

2 See https://www.legacy.com.au/LegacyHistory.

3 Information provided by Mr Rick Cranna, President of Legacy Australia.

4 S. Goulston, 'Talk Given to the NSW Jewish Ex-Servicemen and Women on Armistice Day 1985'. Copy held by Diana Goulston Robinson.

5 See https://www.sydney.edu.au/medicine/museum/mwmuseum/index.php/Postgraduate_Committee_in_Medicine.

6 The number of affected babies born in Australia and New Zealand is believed to be around 150. One of Stan Goulston's radiology colleagues at RPAH, Dr Janet McCredie, later became an international authority on thalidomide and wrote *Beyond Thalidomide: Birth Defects Explained*, published by Royal Society of Medicine Press, 2007.

7 See https://www.tga.gov.au/publication/fifty-years-independent-expert-advice-prescription-medicines and https://www.tga.gov.au/publication/history-therapeutic-goods-regulation-australia.

8 Dr Edgar Thomson served in many other roles as well, including being the Inaugural President of the Royal College of Pathologists of Australasia, head

of the Fairfax Institute of Pathology at the Royal Prince Alfred Hospital and General Superintendent at the same hospital. James C. McAllester and W.D. Refshauge, 'Thomson, Edgar Frederick (1903–1977)', *Australian Dictionary of Biography*, http://adb.anu.edu.au/biography/thomson-edgar-frederick-11852/text21217, published first in hardcopy 2002.

9 See https://www.tga.gov.au/database-adverse-event-notifications-daen.

10 See https://trove.nla.gov.au/version/213895764.

11 S. Goulston, 'Control of Drug Use', *Medical Journal of Australia*, 1981, vol. 1, pp. 166–168.

12 See https://trove.nla.gov.au/newspaper/article/240628622?searchTerm=stanley%20goulston&searchLimits=

13 See https://trove.nla.gov.au/newspaper/article/240701540?searchTerm=stanley%20goulston&searchLimits=

14 Stan Goulston, letter to daughter Diana, 1 March 1987.

12: Poet, Teacher of Medical Humanities and Lover of Nature

1 S. Goulston, 'My New Dignity', *Sun* (Sydney), Sunday 17 August 1930, p. 39.

2 S. Goulston, 'Lights O' Bundanoon', *Sun* (Sydney), 8 June 1930, p. 38.

3 S. Goulston, 'Mowgli', *Sun* (Sydney), 12 October 1930, p. 3.

4 S. Goulston, 'What Does It Mean', *Sun* (Sydney), Sunday 3 August 1930, p. 38.

5 S. Goulston, 'At Watson's Bay', *The Sydneian*, 1930, vol. 280, p. 22.

6 Kenneth Kock, 'The Language of Poetry', *New York Review of Books*, 14 May 1988.

7 Stan Goulston, interview, 2008.

8 The Goulstons were early supporters of Musica Viva in Sydney, a group founded in 1945 by Jewish *émigrés* for the purpose of bringing chamber music to Australia. See https://en.wikipedia.org/wiki/Musica_Viva_Australia.

9 Zara and Tom Selby accompanied them on many occasions. Zara Selby, interview, April 2020.

10 S.J.M. Goulston, *Poetry for Pleasure*, 2007, p. 70.

11 Stan Goulston, letter to daughter Diana, 3 October 1993.

12 As he explained to an interviewer, this was because 'often a word you want is not there'. He used his thesauruses only occasionally for his poems.

13 Excerpts from *Poetry for Pleasure.*

14 The four poems appear in *Poetry for Pleasure*. The poem entitled 'Words and Punctuation Marks' was published in the *Medical Journal of Australia* in 1970. The poem 'Dunkirk', written in 1940 and originally entitled 'Ships Are the Thing – Dunkirk', was published in 1995 (*Medical Journal of Australia*, 1995, vol. 163, nos 11–12, p. 621); 'Life after 80' appeared in 1993 (*Medical Journal of Australia*, 1993, vol. 159, nos 11–12, p. 782); 'Time and Medicine' in 1998 (*Medical Journal of Australia*, 1998, vol. 168, no. 2, p. 87). The latter had been written twenty years earlier, as a reaction to a government decision that general practitioners would be paid on a time basis.

15 These are the combined sentiments of two independent published poets who were invited to read *Poetry for Pleasure*.

16 Kerry Goulston, e-mail to author, March 2020.

17 See https://en.wikipedia.org/wiki/Grace_Perry.

18 Miles Little, interview, 29 April 2020. Dr Little was a regular participant who recalled that sometimes the group would convene at the home of Dr Peter Baume.

19 'Grand Rounds' referred originally to large ward rounds but they are no longer conducted in a ward at the bedside of the patient. Instead they take the form of an educational conference attended by senior and junior medical staff. At Royal Prince Alfred Hospital (RPAH), they formed part of a busy academic programme that filled Friday afternoons and were held from 4 p.m. to 5 p.m. Goulston's poetry Grand Round was part of this programme for several years.

20 The selection of poems for a presentation to the Northern Clinical School of the University of Sydney on 29 June 2000 is held by a daughter. Goulston called his talk 'The Responsibility of a Doctor to His Patient through the Eyes of a Poet'. Poems selected covered talking with the dying, the death of a child, suicide, consent for surgery, and the giving of hope. The intent overall seems to have been to make young doctors more sensitive to the impact of their conversations with patients.

21 S.J.M. Goulston, 'A Selection of Poems Presented by Dr Stanley Goulston to a Meeting of the NSW Society of the History of Medicine', Sydney, 1996.

22 Dr Eric Goulston, letter to his niece Diana, in New York, 1999.

23 Observations recorded by noted virologist, Dr Yvonne Cossart. See https://www.sydney.edu.au/medicine/museum/mwmuseum/index.php/Goulston,_Stanley.

24 Dr Miles Little, interview, 29 April 2020.

25 J. Wright, 'Therapy', in Angela Belli and Jack Coulehan (eds), *Blood and Bone: Poems by Physicians*, 1998.

26 Goulston explained this link with the analogy that 'medicine is all about human understanding of the body, mind, people, and everything else and literature is similar in that respect. It deals with people and events and so on.' Interview, 2008.

27 Stan Goulston, letter to daughter Diana, 31 December 1994.

28 A. Sarzin, *University of Sydney News*, 7 August 1997, vol. 29, no. 17, p. 8.

29 Stan Goulston, letter to daughter Diana, 15 March 1997.

30 'Obituary: Dame Leonie Kramer, a Celebrated Academic and a Potent Conservative Voice', *Sydney Morning Herald*, 21 April 2016.

31 His submission to the Faculty of Medicine forms an appendix to this book. It succinctly outlines his arguments for exposing medical students to literature.

32 In 2003, medical student Arianne Sweeting, now an endocrinologist at RPAH, wrote a long letter of appreciation which Goulston filed among his papers.

33 One student group, which contained several musicians, put on a small concert for Goulston and his wife in appreciation of the course. Sadhana Goulston, interview, 1 May 2020.

34 Tim G., e-mail to Dr Goulston, 23 October 1999.

35 Ibid. Also Arianne Sweeting, letter to Stan Goulston, 2003.

36 S.J.M. Goulston, 'Medical Education in 2001: The Place of Medical Humanities', *Internal Medicine Journal*, 2001, vol. 31, pp. 123–127.

37 A.R. Moore, *The Missing Medical Text: Humane Patient Care*, 1978. In this book, Dr Moore describes his course in detail.

38 Dr Jill Gordon, interview, 6 May 2020.

39 Dr Derek Myers made this prediction in a review of Dr Moore's book, *The Missing Medical Text*. See *Medical Journal of Australia*, 1979, vol. 1, p. 469.

40 J. Gordon, 'New Course in Medical Humanities', *Radius*, October 2003.

41 S. Goulston, 'Attitudes to Retirement', *RACP News*, October 2005, p. 6.

42 Stan Goulston, interview, 2008.

13: Contemplations in the Third Age

1 Stan Goulston, interview, 2008.

2 Ibid.

3 Sadhana Goulston, interview, 1 May 2020.

4 Transcription of a recorded speech given by Wendy Goulston on 13 February 2005. Copy held by Diana Goulston Robinson.

5 Ibid.

6 Stan Goulston, letter to the author, 6 October 2009.

7 S. Goulston, 'Attitudes to Retirement', *RACP News*, October 2005, p. 6.

8 Wendy Goulston, interview, May 2020.

9 Stan Goulston, interview 2008.

Epilogue

1 His second daughter also wrote a eulogy, but because of Jewish protocol was not permitted to deliver it. However, Rabbi Lawrence was able to use much of its content.

2 R. Mulhearn, 'Dr Stanley Goulston, AO, MC, FRACP (1915–2011)', *RACP News*, October 2011, p. 42.

3 J. Lawrence, letter to the Goulston family, letter undated.

4 Emeritus Professor Miles Little, interview, 29 April 2020.

Appendix A: The Life of Dr Eric Goulston (brother of Stanley)

1 Lise Mellor, 'Goulston, Eric', 2008, Faculty of Medicine Online Museum and Archive, University of Sydney, http://sydney.edu.au/medicine/museum/mwmuseum/index.php/Goulston,_Eric.

Appendix B:
'Humane Values in Medical Education: Shaping the Doctor – Literature'

1 S.J.M. Goulston, Submission to the Faculty of Medicine, University of Sydney, 1997. Retyped from the original.

2 General Medical Council, *Tomorrow's Doctors: Recommendations on Undergraduate Education*, 1993.

3 Anthony R. Moore, 'Preface', *The Missing Medical Text: Humane Patient Care*, 1978, p. x.

4 Rita Charon and Peter Williams, 'Introduction', 'The Humanities and Medical Education', *Academic Medicine*, 1995, vol. 70, pp. 758–759.

5 Joanne Trautmann, 'The Wonders of Literature in Medical Education', *Journal of Continuing Education in the Health Professions*, July 1982, vol. 2, no. 3, pp. 23–31 at p. 24.

6 Raymond Carver, 'What the Doctor Said', *A New Path to the Waterfall*, Globe/Atlantic Monthly Press, 1989, quoted by Anne Hunsaker Hawkins, 'Furthermore', *Academic Medicine*, 1994, vol. 69, pp. 278–279.

7 May Sarton, *A Private Mythology*, 'Death of a Psychiatrist', 1966, pp. 97–98.

8 Howard Brody, *Placebos and the Philosophy of Medicine: Conceptual and Ethical Issues*, 1980.

9 Kathryn Montgomery Hunter, *Doctors' Stories: The Narrative Structure of Medical Knowledge*, 1991, pp. 13–14.

10 Robert Coles, *The Call of Stories*, 1989, 'Introduction', pp. xvii–xx.

11 Rodney Hall (ed.), *Michael Dransfield: Collected Poems*, St Lucia, Qld: University of Queensland Press, 1987.

Sources and Bibliography

Interviews and e-mails

In 1990, Dr Stan Goulston was interviewed by Dr Greg Whelan for the archives of the Gastroenterological Society of Australia. Summary of this interview provided by historian Emma Russell.

In 2004, Stan and Jean Goulston gave a joint extended interview to a family member, Diana Goulston Robinson, who was assisted by her daughter Amelia. The transcript of this interview is held by the Goulston family. Throughout this book, this is identified as 'Stan Goulston, interview, 2004' or 'Jean Goulston, interview, 2004'.

In 2008, over several weeks, Lucy Chipkin from the Sydney Jewish Museum interviewed Stan Goulston on six occasions. At times a different daughter was present and when one was there, she participated in the interview. The transcripts are held by the family. In this book, the series of interviews is identified as 'Stan Goulston, interview, 2008'.

Interviews conducted by the author

Dr Alex Bune, April 2020

Emeritus Professor John Chalmers, April 2020

Dr Allan Cooke, April 2020

Dr Jill Gordon, May 2020

Ms Diana Goulston Robinson, April 2020

Dr Kerry Goulston, March 2020

Ms Sadhana Goulston, May 2020

Ms Wendy Goulston, May 2020

Ms Sue Hallenstein (née Goulston), January, May 2020

Mrs Judy Lee, February 2020

Emeritus Professor Steven Leeder, April 2020

Emeritus Professor Miles Little, April 2020

Dr Janet McCredie, May 2020

Dr Bob McRitchie, April 2020

Dr Brian Morgan, May 2020

Dr Jim Rankin, April 2020

Dr Warwick Selby, April 2020

Mrs Zara Selby (née Kingston), April 2020

Dr Arianne Sweeting, April 2020

Dr Greg Whelan, March 2020

E-mails received by the author

Professor John Chalmers, 23 January 2020

Ms Diana Goulston Robinson, 28 April 2020

Dr Kerry Goulston, March–May 2020

Dr Michael Pain, 11 March 2020

Archival sources

Library of the Royal Australasian College of Physicians

Archives of Sydney Grammar School

Records of the Gastroenterological Society of Australia

Unpublished sources

(Unless otherwise specified, these documents are held by the Goulston family.)

A) By/about Dr Eric Goulston (chronologically)

Eric Goulston, 'John Goulston (1869–1961) by Eric Goulston', undated.

Eric Goulston, letter to grandson, Sam Goulston Robinson, undated.

Dr Eric Goulston, letter to his niece, Diana, 1999.

Dr Eric Goulston: 'Wrong Side of Seventy', video including interviews with the three Goulston brothers – Eric, Stan and Roy. Created by Jim Gerrand, 1999.

B) By/about Dr Stan Goulston (chronologically)

Photo albums of Stan Goulston.

Citation for the award of the Military Cross, 10 October 1944.

S. Goulston, unpublished manuscript, 'The Figtree, the Libyan Campaign and the 2/1 Aust Pioneer Battalion'.

S. Goulston, 'Medical History of 2/1st Aust Pioneer Battalion. Medical Chapter.'

Letters of reference concerning Stan Goulston, addressed to the Royal Prince Alfred Hospital, Sydney, 1946

Colonel John H. Anderson, 1946.

Dr Lorimer Dodds, 16 September 1946.

Dr John Halliday, 11 September 1946.

Dr N. Hamilton Fairley, 19 August 1946.

Dr Charles Kellaway, 20 August 1946.

Dr W.P. MacCallum, 24 August 1946.

Dr Kempson Maddox, 18 April 1946.

Dr John McMichael, 2 September 1946.

Dr A.W. Morrow, 18 August 1946.

Dr Sheila Sherlock, August 1946.

Stan Goulston, letter to daughter Diana, 2 April 1977.

Stan Goulston, letter to daughter Diana, 16 October 1977.

S. Goulston, 'Talk Given to the NSW Jewish Ex-Servicemen and Women on Armistice Day, 1985'.

Stan Goulston, letter to daughter Diana, 1 March 1987.

Stan Goulston, letter to daughter Diana, 6 July 1991.

Stan Goulston, letter to daughter Diana, 3 October 1993.

Stan Goulston, letter to daughter Diana, 31 December 1994.

Stan Goulston, letter to daughter Diana, 15 March 1997.

S.J.M. Goulston, 'Humane Values in Medical Education: Shaping the Doctor – Literature', submission to the Faculty of Medicine, University of Sydney, 1997.

Jim Gerrand, *Dr Eric Goulston, 'Wrong Side of Seventy'*, video including interviews with the three Goulston brothers – Eric, Stan and Roy, created 1999. Copy held by Sue and Hal Hallenstein.

Ms Arianne Sweeting, letter to Dr Stan Goulston entitled 'Reflections on Dr Stan Goulston's Literature Option – Semester One 2003'.

Wendy Goulston, transcription of a speech about Stan Goulston, as recorded 13 February 2005. Copy held by Diana Goulston Robinson.

Stan Goulston, letter to Kerry Breen, 6 October 2009. Held by Kerry Breen.

Dr Jim Lawrence, letter to the Goulston family, 2011.

Dr J. Schneeweiss, AM, letter to the Goulston family, 2 September 2011.

Excerpt of a report of the handing-over of a Rats of Tobruk Medal in 2011 from the Australian War Museum.

Published sources

Announcement: 'At Home', *The Hebrew Standard of Australasia*, 3 August 1928, p. 6.

Apple, Raymond, *The Great Synagogue: A History of Sydney's Big Shule*, Sydney: University of New South Wales Press, 2008.

'Board of Censors', *Australian and New Zealand Journal of Medicine*, 1974, vol. 4, no. 2, p. 218.

Boden, R.W., Rankin, J.G., Goulston, S.J. and Morrow, A.W., 'The Liver in Ulcerative Colitis', *Lancet*, 1959, vol. ii, pp. 245–248.

Braithwaite, P., 'The Regimental Medical Officer', *Medical Journal of Australia*, 1943, vol. 1, pp. 137–142.

Breen, K.J., *The Man We Never Knew: Carl de Gruchy – Medical Pioneer*, Faculty of Medicine, University of Melbourne, 2019, p. 99.

Breen, K.J., Cordner, S.M. and Thomson, C.H., *Good Medical Practice: Professionalism, Ethics and Law*, 4th edn, Canberra: Australian Medical Council, 2016.

Brody, Howard, *Placebos and the Philosophy of Medicine: Conceptual and Ethical Issues*, Chicago: University of Chicago Press, 1980.

Buckley, John, *Recollections of the Roving Staff Officer*, Canberra: Department of Defence, 1993.

Cassab, Judy, *Judy Cassab Diaries*, Sydney: Random House, 1995.

'Centenary Convocation', *RPA Magazine*, 1983, Spring edition, pp. 4–5.

'The Centenary Fund', *The Sydneian*, 1957, no. 339, p. 107.

Charon, Rita and Williams, Peter, 'Introduction', 'The Humanities and Medical Education', *Academic Medicine*, 1995, vol. 70, pp. 758–759.

'Chemical Warfare: Compiled under the direction of the Committee on the Survey of War Medicine of the National Health and Medical Research Council', *Medical Journal of Australia*, 1943, vol. 1, pp. 29–32.

'Clinical Meeting at 2/11 Australian General Hospital', *Medical Journal of Australia*, 1942, vol. 2, pp. 470–473.

'Clinical Meeting in the Middle East', *Medical Journal of Australia*, 1942, vol. 2, pp. 14–17.

Cohen, Lysbeth, *Beginning with Esther: Jewish Women in New South Wales from 1788*, Sydney: Ayers & James Heritage Books in association with the Australian Jewish Times, 1987.

Coles, Robert, *The Call of Stories*, Boston: Houghton Mifflin, 1989.

Cooper, E.L., 'Relapsing Fever in Tobruk', *Medical Journal of Australia*, 1942, vol. 1, pp. 635–637.

Cooper, E.L. and Sinclair, A.J.M., 'War Neuroses in Tobruk: A Report on 207 Patients from the Australian Imperial Force Units in Tobruk', *Medical Journal of Australia*, 1942, vol. 2, pp. 73–77.

Crowe, P.J. and Goulston, S., 'Post-gastrectomy Dietary Management', *Medical Journal of Australia*, 1954, vol. 2, pp. 430–433.

'Degree of Doctor of Medicine (Honoris Causa)', [RACP] *Fellowship Affairs Newsletter*, November 1983, vol. 2, no. 4, p. 8.

Devine, J., 'A Note on Desert Sores', *Medical Journal of Australia*, 1943, vol. 2, pp. 261–262.

Devine, John, *The Rats of Tobruk*, Sydney: Angus and Roberston, 1943.

Doherty, M.K., edited by R.L. Russell, *The Life and Times of Royal Prince Alfred Hospital, Sydney, Australia*, Sydney: New South Wales College of Nursing, 1996.

FitzSimons, Peter, *Tobruk*, Pymble, NSW: Harper Collins, 2006.

Freudenberg, Graham, *Churchill and Australia*, Sydney: Pan MacMillan Australia, 2008.

Gallagher, Neil, 'Morrow, Sir Arthur William (Bill) (1903–1977)', *Australian Dictionary of Biography*, National Centre of Biography, Australian National University, http://adb.anu.edu.au/biography/morrow-sir-arthur-william-bill-11178/text19919, published first in hardcopy 2000, accessed online 11 May 2020.

Gallagher, N.D. (ed.), *The A.W. Morrow Unit: 50 Years of Australian Gastroenterology at Royal Prince Alfred Hospital, 1948–1998*, 1998.

Gallagher, N.D. and Goulston, S.J., 'Antibiotic Associated Colitis: In Search of a Cause and Treatment, *Drugs*, 1978, vol. 16, pp. 385–386.

Gallagher, N.D., Goulston, S.J.M., Wyndham, N. and Sir William Morrow, 'The Management of Fulminant Ulcerative Colitis', *Gut*, 1962, vol. 3, pp. 306–311.

General Medical Council, *Tomorrow's Doctors: Recommendations on Undergraduate Education*, London, 1993.

Gordon, J., 'New Course in Medical Humanities', *Radius*, October 2003.

Goulston, E., 'Guerrilla surgery', *Medical Journal of Australia*, 1942, vol. 2, pp. 134–136.

Goulston, K.J., 'A Doctor, a Poet, and Many Other Roles [Obituary]', *Sydney Morning Herald*, 7 October 2011.

Goulston, S./ S.J./ S.J.M., 'At Watson's Bay', *The Sydneian*, 1932, vol. 280, p. 32.

———'Attitudes to Retirement', *RACP News*, October 2005, p. 6.

——— 'Control of Drug Use', *Medical Journal of Australia*, 1981, vol. 1, pp. 166–168.

——— 'A Doctor at War', *Parade* [official organ of the Australian Federation of Jewish Ex-Service Associations], March 1988.

——— 'Dunkirk' [written in 1940 and originally entitled 'Ships Are the Thing – Dunkirk'], *Medical Journal of Australia*, 1995, vol. 163, nos 11–12, p. 621.

——— 'Experience with Infectious Hepatitis at Royal Prince Alfred Hospital, *Medical Journal of Australia*, 1953, vol. 1, pp. 905–913.

——— 'The Influence of the Royal Australasian College of Physicians on Physician Training and Evaluation. 1', *Medical Journal of Australia*, 1974, vol. 1, pp. 203–209.

——— 'The Influence of the Royal Australasian College of Physicians on Physician Training and Evaluation. 2', *Medical Journal of Australia*, 1974, vol. 1, pp. 247–254.

——— 'Ischaemic Colitis', *Medical Journal of Australia*, 1973, vol. 1, pp. 1194–1197.

——— 'Jolly Games Breaking the Stick', *Sun* (Sydney), Sunday 20 April 1930, p. 42.

——— 'Lights O' Bundanoon', *Sun* (Sydney), 8 June 1930, p. 38.

——— 'Life after 80', *Medical Journal of Australia*, 1993, vol. 159, nos 11–12, p. 782.

——— 'The Malaria Frontline. Pioneering Malaria Research by the

Australian Army in World War II' [letter], *Medical Journal of Australia*, 1997, vol. 166, no. 12, p. 672.

——— 'Management of Hiatus Hernia', *Australian and New Zealand Journal of Surgery*, 1956, vol. 26, pp. 101–105.

——— 'Medical Education in 2001: The Place of Medical Humanities', *Internal Medicine Journal*, 2001, vol. 31, pp. 123–127.

——— 'Mowgli', *Sun* (Sydney), 12 October 1930, p. 3.

——— 'My New Dignity', *Sun* (Sydney), Sunday 17 August 1930, p 39.

——— 'The Need for a Medical Liaison Officer in Peace and War', *Medical Journal of Australia*, 1947, vol. 2, pp. 329–332.

——— 'A Personal Appreciation of Dr Vincent McGovern', *Pathology*, 1985, vol. 2, p. 151.

——— *Poetry for Pleasure*, Sydney: ETT Imprint, 2007.

——— 'Recent Advances in Medicine in England', *Medical Journal of Australia*, 1947, vol. 2, pp. 8–10.

——— 'A Regimental Aid Post in Tobruk', *Medical Journal of Australia*, 1942, vol. 1, no. 17, pp. 494–496.

——— 'Time and Medicine', *Medical Journal of Australia*, 1998, vol. 168, no. 2, p. 87.

——— 'The Treatment of Peptic Ulceration', *Medical Journal of Australia*, 1952, vol. 1, pp. 291–293.

——— 'The Value and Limitations of X-ray Examination in Assessing Disease of the Gall-bladder', *Medical Journal of Australia*, 1952, vol. 1, pp. 323–325.

——— 'What Does It Mean', *Sun* (Sydney), 8 June 1930, p. 38.

Goulston, S. and Breen, K., 'Gastroenterology in Australia, 1949–1969', *Postgraduate Medical Journal*, 1970, vol. 46, pp. 210–220.

Goulston, S.J./ S.J.M. and McGovern, V.J., 'Clinical Settings in Pseudomembranous Colitis', *Australian and New Zealand Journal of Medicine*, 1980, vol. 10, pp. 139–145.

——— and McGovern, V.J., *Fundamentals of Colitis*, Oxford; New York: Pergamon Press, 1981.

——— and McGovern, V.J., 'The Nature of Benign Strictures in Ulcerative Colitis', *New England Journal of Medicine*, 1969, vol. 281, pp. 290–295.

——— and McGovern, V.J., 'Pseudo-membranous Colitis', *Gut*, 1965, vol. 6, pp. 207–212.

——— and McGovern, V.J., 'The Value of Rectal Biopsies', *Medical Journal of Australia*, 1972, vol. 1, pp. 1234–1238.

Goulston, S. and Smith, M., 'An Analysis of the Value of Medical Care in a Group of Repatriation Male Duodenal Ulcer Patients', *Australasian Annals of Medicine*, 1955, vol. 4, pp. 255–260.

——— and Smith, M., 'Intrahepatic Biliary Obstruction of Unknown Origin', *Medical Journal of Australia*, 1951, vol. 2, pp. 313–317.

Hassall J., *RPA & Beyond: An Unauthorised Memoir*, Willoughby, NSW: Phillip Mathews Book Publishers, 2010.

Hawkins, Anne Hunsaker, 'Furthermore', *Academic Medicine*, 1994, vol. 69, pp. 278–279.

'The Herbert Webb Prize', *The Sydneian*, 1924, no. 254, p. 42.

Hone, F.R., Keogh, E.V. and Andrew, R., 'Bacillary Dysentery in an Australian Hospital in the Middle East', *Medical Journal of Australia*, 1942, vol. 1, pp. 631–635.

Horan, J., 'Gastroscopy', *Medical Journal of Australia*, 1937, vol. 2, pp. 243–248.

Hunter, Kathryn Montgomery, *Doctors' Stories: The Narrative Structure of Medical Knowledge*, Princeton, New Jersey: Princeton University Press, 1991.

'In Memoriam: Herbert Webb', *The Sydneian*, 1928, no. 266, p. 71.

Johnson, A., 'Obituary. Vincent John McGovern', *Australasian Journal of Dermatology*, 1984, vol. 25, pp. 35–36.

Kock, Kenneth, 'The Language of Poetry', *New York Review of Books*, 14 May 1988.

Lazaridis, K.N. and LaRusso, N.F., 'Primary Sclerosing Cholangitis', *New England Journal of Medicine*, 2016, vol. 375, pp. 1161–1170.

Levi, J.S., 'Danglow, Jacob (1880–1962)', *Australian Dictionary of Biography*, National Centre of Biography, Australian National University, http://adb.anu.edu.au/biography/danglow-jacob-5878/text10001, published first in hardcopy 1981, accessed online 11 May 2020.

——— *Rabbi Jacob Danglow: The Uncrowned Monarch of Australian Jews*, Melbourne: Melbourne University Press, 1995.

Likeman, Robert, *The Thousand Doors: The Australian Doctors at War Series: Vol. Four: The Middle East and Far East 1929–42*, Ultimo, NSW: Halstead Press, 2014, p. 12.

Love, H.R., 'Dyspeptic Symptoms in Soldiers', *Medical Journal of Australia*, 1943, vol. 2, pp. 101–109.

Macdonald, Graham, 'Sands, John Robert (1919–1980)', *Australian Dictionary of Biography*, National Centre of Biography, Australian National University, http://adb.anu.edu.au/biography/sands-john-robert-11612/text20735, published first in hardcopy 2002, accessed online 11 May 2020.

Marshall, S.V., 'Further Aspects of Anaesthesia under Wartime Conditions', *Medical Journal of Australia*, 1943, vol. 2, pp. 83–85.

McAllester, James C. and W.D. Refshauge, 'Thomson, Edgar Frederick (1903–1977)', *Australian Dictionary of Biography*, National Centre of Biography, Australian National University, http://adb.anu.edu.au/biography/thomson-edgar-frederick-11852/text21217, published first in hardcopy 2002, accessed online 11 May 2020.

McCulloch, J.F., 'Anaesthesia under Wartime Conditions', *Medical Journal of Australia*, 1943, vol. 2, pp. 81–83.

McGovern, V.J. and Goulston, S.J., 'Crohn's Disease of the Colon', *Gut*, 1968, vol. 2, pp. 164–176.

McKernan, Michael, *The Strength of a Nation: Six Years of Australians Fighting for the Nation and Defending the Homefront in WWII*, Crows Nest, NSW: Allen & Unwin, 2008.

'Mr John Goulston's Visit Abroad', *The Hebrew Standard of Australasia*, Thursday 12 October 1939, p. 5.

Mistilis, S.P., 'Natural History of Active Chronic Hepatitis. II. Pathology, Pathogenesis and Clinico-pathological Correlation', *Australasian Annals of Medicine*, 1968, November, vol. 17, no. 4, pp. 277–288.

—— 'Pericholangitis and Ulcerative Colitis. I. Pathology, Etiology and Pathogenesis', *Annals of Internal Medicine*, 1965, vol. 63, pp. 1–16.

Mistilis, S.P. and Blackburn, C.R., 'Active Chronic Hepatitis', *American Journal of Medicine*, 1970, April, vol. 48, no. 4, pp. 484–495.

——— and Blackburn, C.R., 'The Treatment of Active Chronic Hepatitis with 6-Mercaptopurine and Azathioprine', *Australasian Annals of Medicine*, 1967, November, vol. 16, no. 4, pp. 305–311.

Mistilis, S.P. and Goulston, S.J.M., 'Liver Disease in Ulcerative Colitis', in B.N. Brooke (ed.), *Recent Advances in Gastroenterology*, London: Churchill, 1965.

Mistilis, S.P., Skyring, A.P. and Blackburn, C.R., 'Natural History of Active Chronic Hepatitis. I. Clinical Features, Course, Diagnostic Criteria, Morbidity, Mortality and Survival', *Australasian Annals of Medicine*, 1968, August, vol. 17, no. 3, pp. 214–223.

Mistilis, S.P., Skyring, A.P. and Goulston, S.J.M., 'Pericholangitis and

Ulcerative Colitis. II. Clinical Aspects', *Annals of Internal Medicine*, 1965, vol. 63, pp. 17–26.

Moore, A.R., *The Missing Medical Text: Humane Patient Care*, Melbourne: Melbourne University Press, 1978.

Moorehead, Alan, *African Trilogy: The North African Campaign, 1940–43*, UK: Cassell, 1998.

'More on the Rats of Tobruk Medal', Numismatic Bibliomania Society e-newsletter, *The E-Sylum*, 2011, vol. 14, April 17, article 14.

Morlet, C., 'With the Australian Army Medical Corps in Two Sieges: Anzac and Tobruk', *Medical Journal of Australia*, 1943, vol. 2, pp. 221–224.

Morson, B., 'Muscle Abnormality in Ulcerative Colitis', *New England Journal of Medicine*, 1969, vol. 281, pp. 325–326.,

Mulhearn. R., 'Dr Stanley Goulston AO, MC, FRACP (1915–2011)', *RACP News*, October 2011, p. 42.

'News and Notes of Old Sydneians', *The Sydneian*, 1942, no. 308, p. 62.

Niall, Brenda, *Judy Cassab: A Portrait*, Sydney: Allen & Unwin, 2005.

'Obituary: Dame Leonie Kramer, a Celebrated Academic and a Potent Conservative Voice', *Sydney Morning Herald*, 21 April 2016.

'Obituary: Mr Hyman Goulston', *Sydney Morning Herald*, 24 November 1930, p. 11.

'Old Sydneians on Active Service', *The Sydenian*, 1940, no. 303, p. 75.

Osborn, Gordon, *The Pioneers: Unit History of the 2nd/1st Australian Pioneer Battalion, Second AIF*, Beverly Hills, NSW: M.D. Herron, 1988.

'Painting of Mr John Goulston', *The Hebrew Standard of Australasia*, Thursday 13 January 1949, p. 4.

Plueckhahn, V.D., 'Not an Armchair Pathologist – Inaugural John Perry Memorial Oration', *Pathology*, 1977, vol. 9, pp. 1–11.

'Portrait Marks Gastro Transition, *Pacemaker – Staff News Sheet of the Royal Prince Alfred Hospital*, 1983, November, vol. 14, no. 2, p. 2.

'Program of the Ballet and Music Concert of the Palestine Orchestra, Tel Aviv', 26 November 1941. Held by Diana Goulston Robinson.'

Rankin, J.G., Boden, R.W., Goulston, S.J.M. and Morrow, A.W., 'The Liver in Ulcerative Colitis. Treatment of Pericholangitis with Tetracycline', *Lancet*, 1959, vol. ii, pp. 1110–1112.

Rankin, J.G., Goulston, S.J.M., Boden, R.W. and Morrow, A.W., 'Fulminant Ulcerative Colitis', *Quarterly Journal of Medicine*, 1960, vol. 29, pp. 375–389.

'Rat Medal. Pride of Tobruk', *Cairns Post*, 8 January 1942, p. 1.

Royal Prince Alfred Hospital: 125 Year Anniversary Book, Royal Prince Alfred Hospital, 2007, pp. 127–148.

Russell, E. and Sheedy, K., *A Passion for the Gut: The Evolution of Gastroenterology in Australia*, Sydney: Gastroenterological Society of Australia, 2009, p. 9.

Sarton, May, *A Private Mythology*, 'Death of a Psychiatrist', New York: W.W. Norton, 1966.

Sarzin, A., *University of Sydney News*, 7 August 1997, vol. 29, no. 17, p. 8.

'School Notes', *The Sydneian*, 1929, no. 269, p. 21.

'School Training: Democracy and Education', *Sydney Morning Herald,* Saturday 13 December 1930, p. 15.

Sircus, W. 'Milestones in the Evolution of Endoscopy: A Short History', *Journal of the Royal College of Physicians of Edinburgh*, 2003, vol. 33, pp. 124–134.

Smith, E.R. and Goulston, S.J., 'Antibiotic-induced Diarrhoea', *Drugs*, 1975, vol. 10, pp. 329–332.

'Sydney Grammar School. Governor's Address', *Sydney Morning Herald*, Saturday 14 December 1929, p. 22.

Teale, Ruth, 'Schlink, Sir Herbert Henry (1883–1962)', *Australian Dictionary of Biography*, National Centre of Biography, Australian National University, http://adb.anu.edu.au/biography/schlink-sir-herbert-henry-8359/text14551, published first in hardcopy 1988, accessed online 11 May 2020.

'"Tobruk Rat" Medal', *Sydney Morning Herald*, Tuesday 30 December 1941, p. 9.

'Those Who Serve', *The Hebrew Standard of Australasia*, Thursday 18 February 1943, p. 4.

Trautmann, Joanne, 'The Wonders of Literature in Medical Education', *Journal of Continuing Education in the Health Professions*, July 1982, vol. 2, no. 3, pp. 23–31.

'A Tribute to John Goulston', *The Great Synagogue Congregational Journal*, November 1961, p. 5.

Tyers, T.L., 'A New Method of Radiological Localization of Foreign Bodies', *Medical Journal of Australia*, 1942, vol. 1, pp. 493–494.

'Vale – Dr Stan Goulston', *Pioneer News – The Official Organ of 2/1 and 2/2 Pioneer Battalions Association*, November 2011, p. 4.

Walsh, G.P., 'Bushell, Philip Howard (1879–1954)', *Australian Dictionary of Biography*, National Centre of Biography, Australian National University, http://adb.anu.edu.au/biography/bushell-philip-howard-5439/text9233, published first in hardcopy 1979, accessed online 11 May 2020.

Wilmot, Chester, *Tobruk 1941*, Penguin Books, 1944.

——— *Tobruk 1941, Capture – Siege – Relief*, Angus & Robertson Ltd, 1945.

Winton, R., *Why the Pomegranate? A History of the Royal College of Physicians of Australasia*, Sydney: RACP, 1988, p. 32.

Wiseman, J.C. (ed.), *To Follow Knowledge: A History of Examinations, Continuing Education and Specialist Affiliations of the Royal Australasian College of Physicians*, Sydney: RACP, 1988.

Wright, J., 'Therapy', in Angela Belli and Jack Coulehan (eds), *Blood and Bone: Poems by Physicians*, Iowa City: University of Iowa Press, 1998.

Web sources

http://aagps.nsw.edu.au/about/history/

http://adb.anu.edu.au/biography/bushell-philip-howard-5439/text9233

http://adb.anu.edu.au/biography/morrow-sir-arthur-william-bill-11178/text19919

http://adb.anu.edu.au/biography/sands-john-robert-11612/text20735

https://ahha.asn.au/about-sidney-sax

https://commons.wikimedia.org/wiki/Category:Johan_de_Witt_(ship,_1920)

https://en.wikipedia.org/wiki/Commonwealth_Day

https://en.wikipedia.org/wiki/Grace_Perry

https://en.wikipedia.org/wiki/Musica_Viva_Australia

https://en.wikipedia.org/wiki/RMS_Orion

https://en.wikipedia.org/wiki/RMS_Queen_Elizabeth#Second_World_War

https://en.wikipedia.org/wiki/Scipio_Africanus

https://en.wikipedia.org/wiki/Sheila_Sherlock

https://en.wikipedia.org/wiki/Sir_John_McMichael

https://en.wikipedia.org/wiki/Sydney_Grammar_School

https://en.wikisource.org/wiki/The_Times/1914/Arts/For_the_Fallen

https://en.wikipedia.org/wiki/William_Slim,_1st_Viscount_Slim

http://guides.naa.gov.au/safe-haven/chapter7/index.aspx

http://munksroll.rcplondon.ac.uk/Biography/Details/3556

https://nthsyddem-p.schools.nsw.gov.au/about-our-school.html

https://royalsociety.org/grants-schemes-awards/awards/copley-medal/

http://sydney.edu.au/medicine/museum/mwmuseum/index.php/Morrow,_Sir_Arthur_William

https://trove.nla.gov.au/list?id=124294

https://trove.nla.gov.au/newspaper/article/240628622?searchTerm=stanley%20goulston&searchLimits=

https://trove.nla.gov.au/version/213895764

https://www.165macquariestreet.com.au/

https://www.bsg.org.uk/about/history-of-the-bsg/

https://www.coinbooks.org/esylum/

https://www.defence.gov.au/adc/adfj/Documents/issue_75/75_1989_Mar_Apr.pdf

https://www.gastro.org/about-aga/about-us

https://www.geni.com/people/John-Goulston/6000000041370933612

https://www.gov.uk/guidance/medals-campaigns-descriptions-and-eligibility

https://www.holocaust.com.au/australia-and-the-european-theatres-of-war/

https://www.independent.co.uk/arts-entertainment/obituary-professor-bryan-brooke-1175817.html

https://www.independent.co.uk/news/obituaries/obituary-sir-francis-avery-jones-1159805.html

https://www.legacy.com.au/LegacyHistory

https://www.mapmycareer.health.nsw.gov.au/Pages/specialty-details.aspx?specialty=50§ion=ms

https://www.nswjbd.org/about-us/

https://www.nytimes.com/1983/07/30/obituaries/dr-burrill-b-crohn-99-an-expert-on-diseases-of-the-intestinal-tract.html

https://www.pymblelc.nsw.edu.au/

https://www.racp.edu.au/about/college-roll/college-roll-bio/bye-william-alick

https://www.racp.edu.au/about/college-roll/college-roll-bio/greenaway-i-sir-i-thomas-moore

https://www.sydney.edu.au/medicine/museum/mwmuseum/index.php/Blackburn,_Charles_Ruthven_Bickerton

https://www.sydney.edu.au/medicine/museum/mwmuseum/index.php/Goulston,_Stanley

https://www.tga.gov.au/database-adverse-event-notifications-daen

https://www.tga.gov.au/publication/fifty-years-independent-expert-advice-prescription-medicines

https://www.tga.gov.au/publication/history-therapeutic-goods-regulation-australia

https://www.theguardian.com/australia-news/2019/may/03/college-of-physicians-under-investigation-after-years-of-reported-dysfunction

Index

For subjects followed by asterisk (*), see related image(s) in Plates section, between p. 68 and p. 69.

Acknowledgements

I first met Dr Stanley Goulston across the examiners' table when I sat the clinical examination for Membership of the Royal Australasian College of Physicians (MRACP) in Brisbane in September 1968. He was one of the college censors. Four months later, as a fifth-year medical graduate, I took up my appointment as Registrar to the A.W. Morrow Department of Gastroenterology at the Royal Prince Alfred Hospital (RPAH) in Sydney and met Dr Goulston in circumstances less stressful for me. In my eighteen months at RPAH, I found him to be exactly as collectively described by the people interviewed for this book. Small things about his thoroughness and thoughtfulness stick in my mind. One was his insistence on viewing the X-ray films of any patient under his care – a practice that I naturally copied. He did this not because he thought that he knew more than the excellent radiologists with whom he worked, but because, knowing his patients well, he was more aware of what he was searching for – and if the X-rays had come from elsewhere, he needed to ensure that they were of adequate quality. A second small thing was his desire to help trainees to learn, as shown when he went out of his way to find me so that he could demonstrate to me my first case of pseudomembranous colitis.

Thus my first acknowledgment is to state that I came to writing this biography as one of his disciples. This did not stop me enquiring about any negative impacts that Dr Goulston may have had on people with whom he worked. This resulted in just one small hint of dissatisfaction, when a former trainee reported that he complained to Goulston that a successor trainee had not adequately acknowledged the former trainee's earlier contributions to a clinical research publication; the trainee was expecting sympathy and did not receive any. However, that small hiccough did not diminish the deep regard that he had for Dr Goulston.

More directly related to the writing of this account, I must primarily acknowledge the wonderful assistance that I received during my research from Stan Goulston's four daughters – Diana, Wendy, Sue (and her husband, Hal Hallenstein) and Sadhana – and from Stan's nephew, Dr Kerry Goulston, also a gastroenterologist. They all gave their time for interviews, went out of their way to find valuable material for me, and read and corrected as necessary the details in draft chapters. The bulk of the research and writing was done during the Covid-19 virus pandemic and so most of our contact was by telephone and e-mail. Nevertheless the warmth in those communications was what one might expect from the offspring and relatives of Jean and Stan Goulston. I also want to acknowledge the foresight of the extended family when interviews with Stan and Jean (2004) and with Stan (2008) were recorded and transcribed. These were undertaken for the family archives but proved to be a 'treasure trove' for an unanticipated biographer.

As Stan Goulston lived to the age of ninety-six and died in 2011, there were no contemporaries to interview and few of his early trainees were contactable. Nevertheless there were many people who knew him well, professionally and/or personally, or whose careers were influenced by contact with him, who were pleased to be interviewed or to contribute by e-mail. In alphabetical order, they were: Dr Alex Bune, Emeritus Professor John Chalmers, Dr Allan Cooke, Dr Jill Gordon, Mrs Judy Lee, Emeritus Professor Stephen Leeder, Emeritus Professor Miles Little, Dr Janet McCredie, Dr Bob McRitchie, Dr Brian Morgan, Dr Michael Pain, Dr Jim Rankin, Dr Warwick Selby, Mrs Zara Selby, Dr Arianne Sweeting and Dr Greg Whelan. I thank them sincerely for their generosity and valuable input.

Historian Ms Emma Russell kindly provided information gathered when she and her colleague wrote the history of the Gastroenterological Society of Australia (GESA). Their history also proved valuable to me.

Archivists and librarians are essential resource people for biographers and I thank Ms Charlotte McColl, Archivist at Sydney Grammar School and Ms Karen Myers, Librarian at the RACP for their assistance. Although not an archivist, Mr Rick Cranna, chairman of Legacy Australia, generously sought information for me from the files of the Sydney Legacy office. Dr Geoff McCaughan gave me a copy of the history of the A.W. Morrow Department of Gastroenterology, where he is the current Director, and helped to find other information. The President of GESA, Dr Simone Strasser (who is also a staff member of the A.W. Morrow Department) and Ms Fiona Bailey, Chief Executive Officer of GESA, helped to track down information for me.

Other colleagues and friends on whom I prevailed where additional information or special knowledge was required included: Dr Ted Heffernan, Mr Barry Breen, Dr James King, OAM, Dr Katrina Watson, OAM, Mr Ian Frank, AM and Ms Theanne Walters. I especially thank Ms Brenda Niall, AO and Dr Katrina Watson, who kindly provided very helpful feedback on an entire draft manuscript. I thank photographer, Mr Michael Wearne, who travelled to take the excellent photographs of the Rats of Tobruk medal and related mementoes.

I thank the following organisations that gave permission to reproduce material: the Sydney Grammar School Archives, the Faculty of Medicine at the University of Sydney, the Royal Australasian College of Physicians, John Wiley & Sons publisher of the *Medical Journal of Australia*, and Mr Tom Thomson of ETT Imprint, publisher of *Poetry for Pleasure*. Every effort was made to identify who held the copyright for the poem by Dr J. Wright titled 'Therapy', published in *Blood and Bone: Poems by Physicians* edited by Angela Belli and Jack Coulehan, University of Iowa Press, Iowa City, 1998, but three organisations contacted were unable to assist.

I am indebted to Emeritus Professor Miles Little, a colleague and friend to Stan Goulston, for writing a beautiful and perceptive Foreword for the book.

Last, I wish to thank Mr Nick Walker and his wonderful team at Australian Scholarly Publishing for yet again being so easy to work with and doing an excellent job on the design and production of the book.

www.ingramcontent.com/pod-product-compliance
Ingram Content Group Australia Pty Ltd
76 Discovery Rd, Dandenong South VIC 3175, AU
AUHW020137130726
429791AU00003B/88

9 781922 454171